ULTIMATE
MIND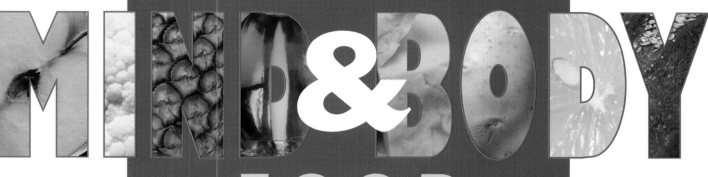&BODY
FOOD

For Healthy Living

BRIDGET JONES

Published in 2002 by Caxton Editions
20 Bloomsbury Street
London WC1B 3JH
a member of the Caxton Publishing Group

© 2002 Caxton Publishing Group

Designed and produced for Caxton Editions
by Open Door Limited, Rutland, UK
Editing: Vanessa Morgan
Typesetting: Jane and Richard Booth
Colour separation: GA Graphics, Stamford, UK

Title: Ultimate Mind and Body Food
ISBN: 1 84067 242 0

Printed and bound by CTPS

ULTIMATE MIND&BODY FOOD

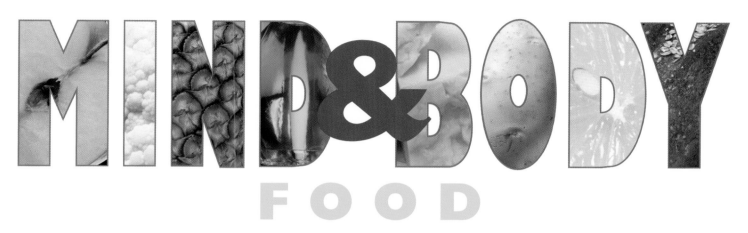

For Healthy Living

BRIDGET JONES

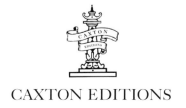

CAXTON EDITIONS

CONTENTS

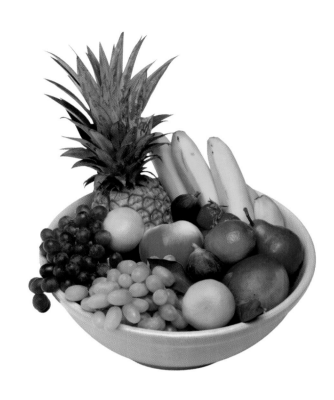

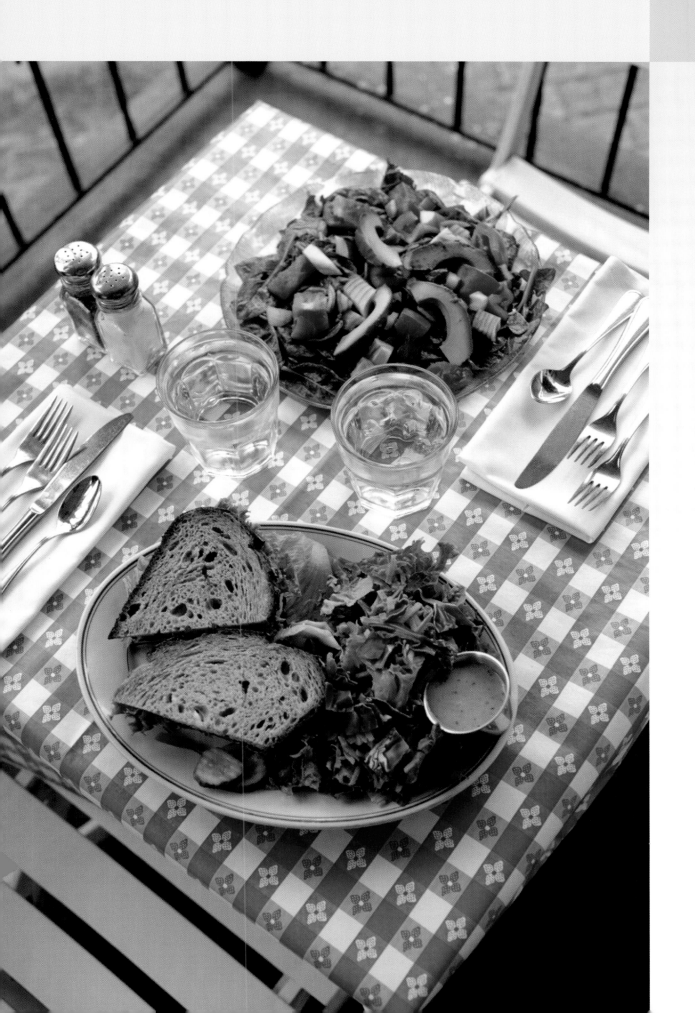

FOOD FOR THOUGHT

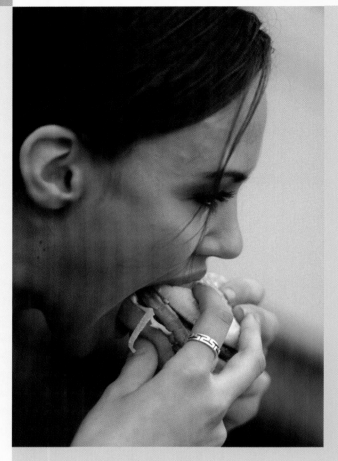

The choice of what, how, when and where to eat is probably one of the broadest for such a basic activity. Decisions about eating at home are mind-boggling: there is an incalculable range of ingredients and products in supermarkets; there are specialist food shops or mail-order options; or cooking is not necessary with the different take-away food options (and because many deliver to the door, there is no need to leave the house to buy the food). Eating out is a commonplace alternative, with options ranging from traditional little eateries to sophisticated restaurants and fashion-focused bars or cafés.

Food has a high profile in the media. It is displayed as a practical subject and for its entertainment value on television or in journals. Diet is the focus for serious discussion and writing on nutrition, social or cultural issues. Take your pick and form an opinion on almost anything from produce that is likely to make you healthy or slowly kill you, to almost-ready dishes to turn you into a wonder chef or keep you ahead of the latest food trends. All this information must promote awareness, satisfaction and ultimate diet fulfilment – or does it?

Life seems to have become ridiculously complicated as we run around in ever-decreasing circles juggling work, family, social and leisure commitments, and everything about eating seems to have joined the fraught spiral. We have so many options that deciding what to eat can be a problem, especially when we are offered conflicting information from all angles. Beyond its function as fuel for life, food plays many complex roles, some we are aware of and others that are almost built into our make up. In western society we do not 'eat to live' in the survival sense.

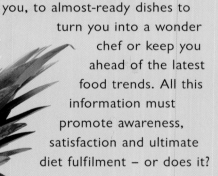

FOOD FOR THOUGHT

Eating:

satisfaction or suspicion?

Barely fifty years ago, eating patterns were largely governed by the seasonal availability of fresh foods. Those who could afford to indulge in expensive and 'exotic' ingredients or eat out in smart restaurants had the advantage of greater flexibility, but the majority of food experiences were limited. However, the culinary world was on the cusp of a major change, already underway in the research and development of food production and manufacturing – even if it was largely curtained from the consumer.

Changing lifestyles, male/female roles and family patterns have turned the simple things in life upside down compared to the expectations of previous generations. Lifestyle is an issue within which everything has to have a function; and the function of everything is open to analysis. The pace of modern living and the incredible number of choices on every level mean assessing and evaluating all options.

Eating exists on levels that have never before been so widely and openly acknowledged. It is no longer a case of regular menus for family breakfast and dinner with packed lunches in between; Saturday lunch and Sunday dinner. People now expect more of food.

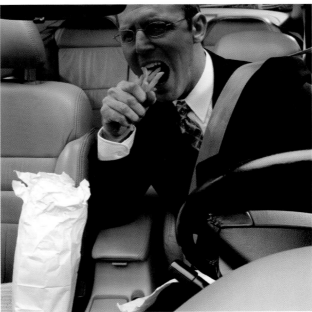

Ultimately, this has not led to satisfaction but to suspicion. We all worry about food, diet and eating in some way. Food shopping is time consuming and stressful. There may be occasional relaxing interludes looking for non-essential items, but the majority of supermarket shopping is noisy, impersonal, time-consuming, fraught with selection decisions, and pitted with possibilities for overspending.

For many, the business of everyday eating can become yet another source of stress and concern in an overworked life. The opposite should be true.

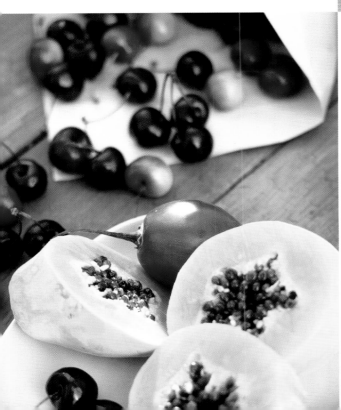

Turning the tables: a positive approach

In this twenty-first century dietary jungle, re-discovering the essence of good eating is not as difficult as it may seem. Food is more closely linked to health than to sustenance. And 'health' no longer isolates the physical from the mental: achieving a sense of wellbeing has emerged as distinct from, but vital to, health. The link between mind and body is broadly acknowledged at all levels and through all stages in life. Over a decade, in western society, the concern has moved from one for good basic nutrition through extremes of healthy diet, then on to balanced eating and to re-establishing the overall importance of food.

Diet choices and meal occasions can be excellent antidotes to the pace of everyday life. Making the right choices are important to relieve one possible source of stress. Sorting out a positive approach to food is the first step in the right direction.

Exploring the way food works on more than a physical level brings several benefits. It is the ideal opportunity to sort out the plethora of information with which we are bombarded by food manufacturers and sellers. It is a good way of getting rid of doubts about quality and taking a personal stand. Taking control of your food purchasing and eating habits empowers you to make the most of your diet and to share this with others around you.

Focusing on food, cooking and eating as one of the most positive aspects of everyday life is truly liberating. Instead of dancing to the tune of food manufacturers selling products that are supposedly 'quick' or 'healthy'

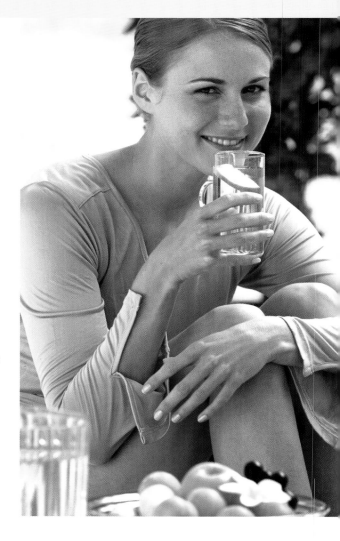

alternatives, discovering simple solutions in basic ingredients is exciting and inspiring. Rather than being caught up in a spiral of dieting and overeating, establishing a moderate eating pattern sets you free from the weight-chasing and meal-missing. Taking personal responsibility for an overall sense of wellbeing is enlightening and re-vitalizing.

Another exhilarating aspect of appreciating food in every sense is the sharing of what you discover with others. Cooking for friends and family and sharing meals is a very positive way of nurturing relationships.

A practical approach: using this book

The chapters that follow highlight the ways in which food influences our everyday lives. Each section explores one topic with the intention of provoking personal opinion. Then there are suggestions for introducing practical everyday improvements. Understanding our own response to food comes first, followed by a reminder that cooking and eating meals can be a caring and enjoyable thing to do. The idea of using different ingredients and cooking methods to nurture a positive approach is important. The role of cooking and eating in daily life leads on to the topic of achieving harmony and a sense of wellbeing.

Recipes created to meet different mental needs follow in five chapters. These include suggestions for initial detoxifying of the system before embarking on a new approach to food.

These are followed by dishes for calming and soothing, or for achieving vitality. Exploring the idea of restoratives and recognizing the need for comfort and reassurance follow.

There is nothing difficult or demanding about the suggestions and recipes. Use the ideas and dishes as a basis on which to build your own ideas and confidence in selecting foods that are best suited to your mental, as well as your physical, needs.

Cooking should be a positive, therapeutic and rewarding activity and an expression of care and love. Feed your mind as well as your body for a positive physical and mental outlook.

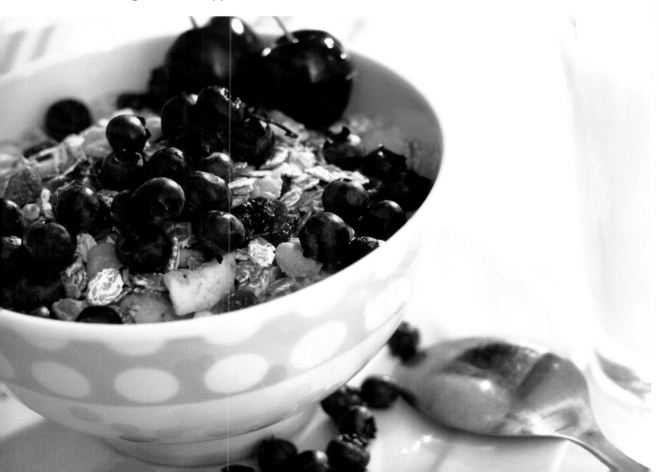

EXPLORING EATING:
IN RESPONSE TO FOOD

We eat to live – or do we? We have to eat to provide our bodies with the fuel they need for survival, activity, growth and repair. These days, in Western society we do far more than just eat to live, as food and eating occasions have become more than a basic necessity. Once hunger pangs and the need for nourishment are fulfilled, appetite is a complex, flexible and changeable sensation. Eating is a naturally enjoyable experience but it can be changed and corrupted by all sorts of influences and pressures. Shopping for food and cooking are activities that are fundamentally satisfying and positive – enjoyable or fun, even – but they are also affected by the pressures of modern living. In this crazy, no-time-to-spare society, it seems that all of a sudden, meals and eating – things that had always felt positive and enjoyable – have gathered black clouds of mixed feelings, or problems, that hover above or close by.

If you identify with these sentiments or recognize any of the symptoms of food stress, take a breather to rediscover one of the most positive, natural and beneficial activities for life-long energy, vitality and wellbeing. Forget cooking chores and focus on food therapy.

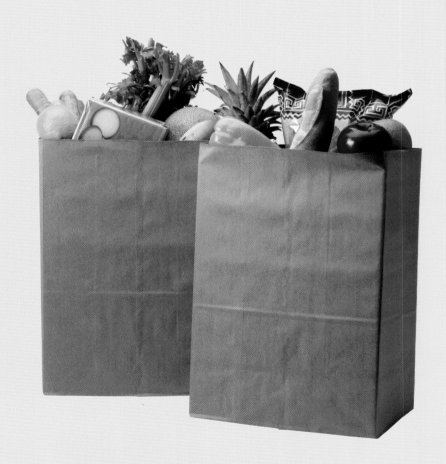

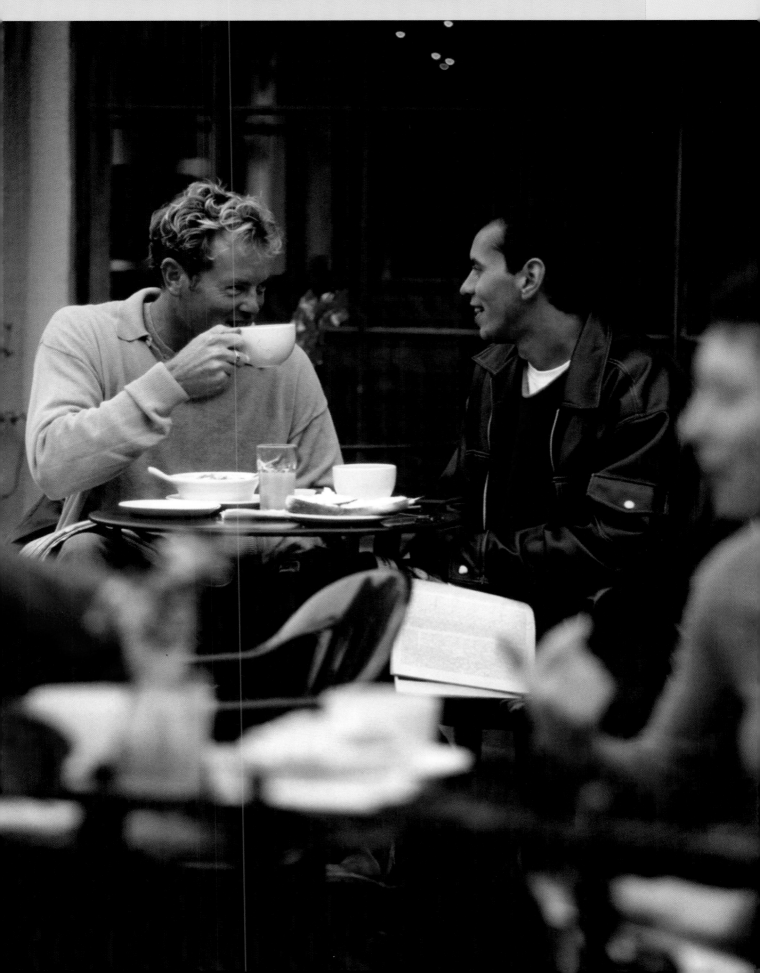

Which foods and why?

Moving on from negative ideas and making the most of the good things in life sometimes means understanding the ways in which we interact with everyday events. Exploring our natural responses to food, and the ways in which contemporary influences make shopping, cooking and eating what it is today, is a good starting point for focusing on the good things and overcoming any bad associations or impressions. From our very first experiences of food to the mass of advertising information we absorb daily, all sorts of influences colour our choices and eating habits. Childhood experiences of eating stay with us into adulthood, although we may not even be aware of them. Similar impressions are collected throughout adult life, either consciously or unconsciously.

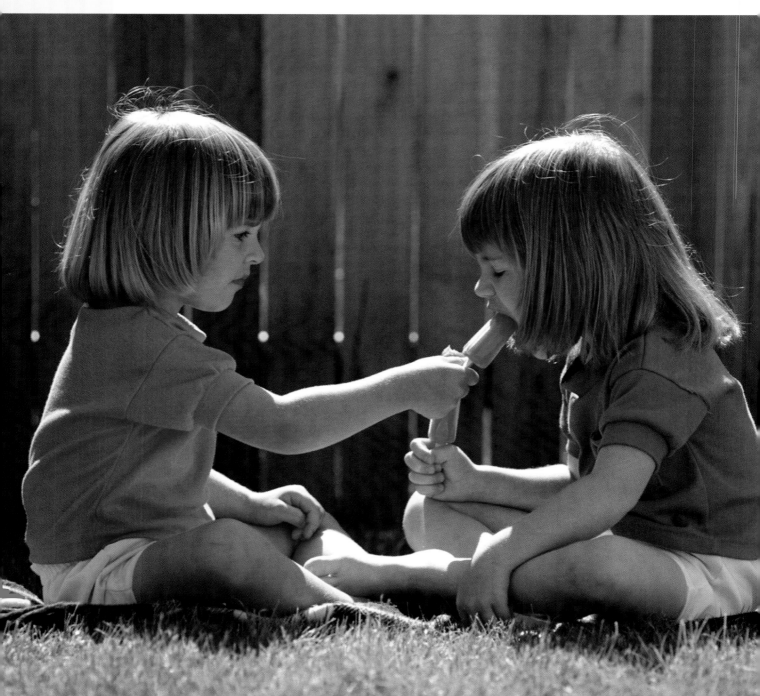

Personal Impressions

- Good or bad childhood associations with foods or eating situations influence the way we 'feel' about foods. In some cases we refuse to sample foods as adults that we took a dislike to in childhood – being encouraged to taste something we thought we disliked can be a great surprise when we realise we do like it after all. The old-fashioned associations with school dinners were often as much with the discipline, serving and eating circumstances as with the food itself.

- Children may reject or eat food because of the influence of others and wanting to mimic people they admire. Such imitative behaviour within a family group can establish life-long beliefs in likes or dislikes. For example, if you never eat a particular food throughout your childhood and teenage years simply because your mother does not like or cook it, then you may well assume an automatic dislike for that food item in adulthood. Unless this is challenged, it can continue throughout life.

- Bad childhood associations between food and people are often difficult to shed. For example, a dislike of a certain ingredient can result from always being given this when visiting someone we did not like. Conversely, being offered food at the house of a favourite relative or neighbour creates a positive link that is likely to survive into adulthood.

- Punishment or reward associations are often linked to food – being made to sit at a table until something had been eaten completely, or receiving other foods as a reward for being good.

- Negative associations with food situations are not necessarily related to taste alone. They may also be linked to smells or eating circumstances. For example, cooking smells or the use of particular table napkins, linen or even lighting can all trigger negative responses to food.

- Dishes or foods associated with happy occasions have positive associations.

- Positive associations with eating situations and ambience can trigger good responses – but sometimes the anticipation is better than the reality. We all remember with affection certain meals that we cooked as students, or dishes we sampled while on holiday, yet when they are recreated they are somehow disappointing.

- Types of food eaten during sad periods can induce negative associations. Eating patterns while we are in a state of personal trauma, such as divorce, bereavement or unemployment, may always be regarded as unpleasant. Very strong links of this type can be difficult to shake off, especially if we are not entirely aware of them. For example, a row between a couple over a dinner table, or family arguments at meal times can have a lasting, negative impression on a whole range of meal, food or eating situations – even though the real impact may be on a subliminal level.

Social and External Influences

- Advertising and lifestyle images influence choice. If an advertisement for a food or product projects an appealing image, it encourages us to try the product.

- Social influences and peer pressure make a great impact, particularly during vulnerable phases when we are keen to establish a social position. Something as simple as eating the same type of food as our contemporaries may be important.

- Children are particularly vulnerable to peer pressure. For example, having the right snack or packed lunch is important if they are to be accepted within their own group. Parents are as aware of this as the children.

- Family pressures can mean that we raise or lower standards or change our attitude to food. Husbands, wives, partners or children can all exert powerful pressure that influences opinions.

- Food scares can make a lasting impression – it is always a good idea to follow through the information and check its validity. Some of the more sensational stories are often short and alarming without being well balanced.

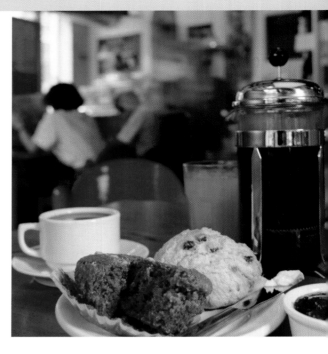

Diet and lifestyle: pace and race

Advances in science and technology have led us to work our bodies mentally into the ground, while reducing the levels of continuous, gentle exercise that benefitted previous generations. We experience stress more widely, to a greater and more prolonged extent, and we are less fit than our parents and grandparents. Our diets contain far more synthetic ingredients and highly processed foods than ever before. Growing concern with the wear and tear that results from our frantic pace of life is gradually making everyone aware of the need for balance. Even those with the minimum interest in eating cannot ignore the fact that there is renewed focus on the traditional acceptance and understanding of a link between what we eat and our health – not just physical health but an overall sense of mind and body harmony. Food can help to balance our mental and physical health once we recognise the ways in which it works, and learn how to relax into food therapy.

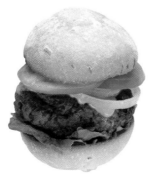

Family ideals: contemporary roles and food choice

We have moved on from the 1950s image of family life – an apron-clad mother waving a duster with one hand, whisking up a cake with the other and running the house to the tune of three meals a day. Meanwhile, father puts his feet up with the paper, waiting for dinner as the children, in woolly dressing gowns, sip milky drinks and nibble biscuits before bed.

Contemporary roles may not be as wildly different as we imagine but they are definitely more flexible and variable. The woman is quite likely to work part- or full-time and the man is less likely to put his feet up waiting for dinner. The household may be a one-parent set-up rather than couple based; today's youngsters exert infinitely more influence than children of the 'fifties. Individuals within the household, young or adult, express their opinions on what they want to eat, where and when, and are more likely to eat separately.

Whereas the 'fifties family always sat down together to eat certain meals, the twenty-first century household is far less likely to meet around the meal table on a daily basis.

Women may be playing different parts but they are still the starting point for decisions on what the family eats. Women still take responsibility for shopping and getting meals on the table. Other adults exert their influence next, followed by children. Putting together meals that will be eaten, rather than rejected, is more important in influencing choice than is the hype on healthy eating. As a whole, and particularly within families, familiar foods are the first choice and they are usually linked to traditional styles. Although serving known main ingredients with unusual sauces or accompaniments may be acceptable, there is a tendency to avoid anything too strange as the main part of the meal.

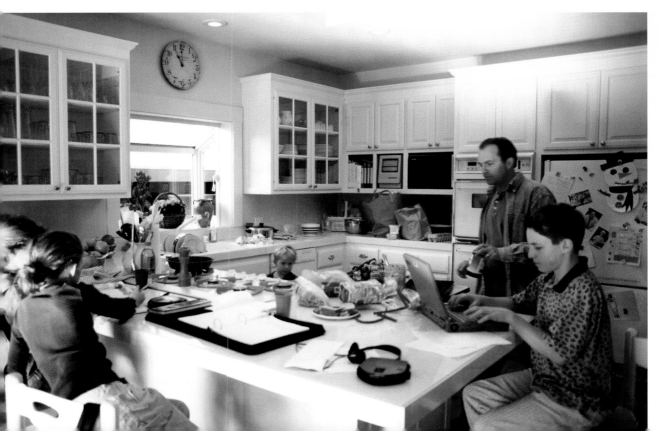

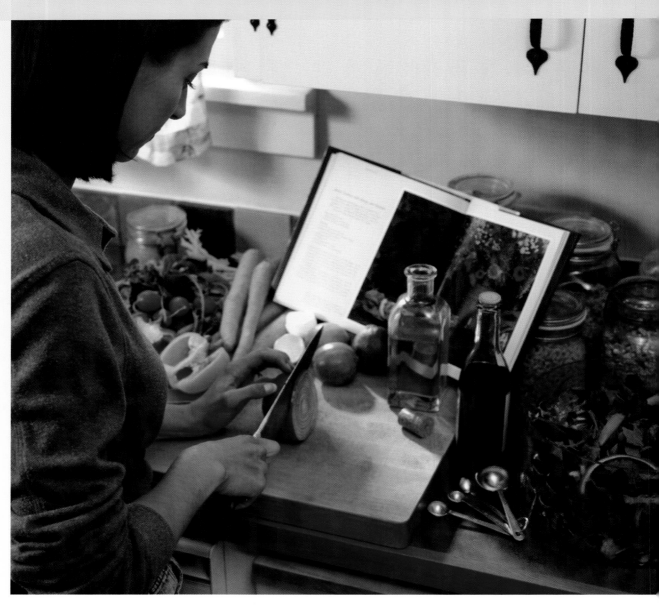

Food fashions and obsessions

It is incredible that eating has reached the point where it can be anything to anyone. Food has become fashionable in such a way that we often spend more time reading about it or watching programmes on the subject than we do selecting ingredients, cooking and eating. There is an almost unreal obsession with discussing, checking and fretting over what a 'healthy' diet should contain, to the extent that there is no time to concentrate on basic, simple cooking.

Instead of always encouraging a positive approach, eating fashions and cooking as entertainment have become destructive for many people. Cooking seems to have become complicated: there is an image of multi-faceted dishes evolving from complicated recipes, and always presented in immaculate condition. Everything seems to be well seasoned with the sort of flamboyant style, humour or entertainment value that is as likely to turn off as many as it attracts.

Somewhere along the line, the idea of balancing straightforward, simple and beneficial everyday cooking with a personal desire to be more adventurous seems to have been overlooked. As a result, many have dismissed cooking as something too difficult to cope with on all but rare occasions. Restaurant meals, bar snacks, take-away foods and ready meals replace many home-cooked meals.

Seriously unhealthy obsessions with the choice of food and diet are not uncommon. Images of unrealistically slim women have encouraged whole generations to follow ridiculously limited diets. Eating disorders have become more common, and are found in men as well as women; they are also evident in children.

Extensive negative publicity about food, eating and cooking has, in some cases, encouraged disproportionate preoccupations with allergies, synthetic ingredients and the potential for food poisoning. While these are all serious concerns, ones that we should be addressing by eating a higher proportion of natural ingredients generated to high quality,

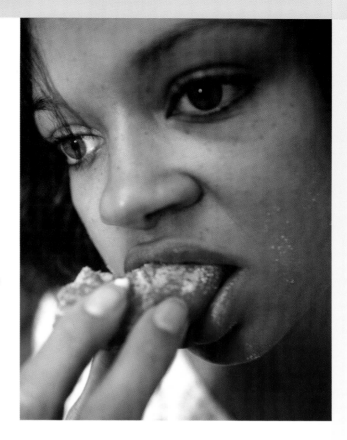

for those who have come to regard food and eating as a 'problem' they can become a real focus for stress.

In a world so obsessed with image and lifestyle, food and eating has become another fashion accessory to flaunt or flap about. Among teenagers and younger groups, it is not considered 'cool' to eat unfashionable foods. In young adults, sharing the same food fears and shopping for the same particular types of ingredients is common within groups. Being 'too busy to cook' is a popular trend across a broad spectrum of age groups. Sharing hearsay and opinions on so-called food allergies (not professionally diagnosed or assessed) provides mutual support for cutting out whole groups of ingredients (with the loss of the nutrients they provide), without taking a healthy perspective on balanced eating or exploring the source of problems properly before changing the diet.

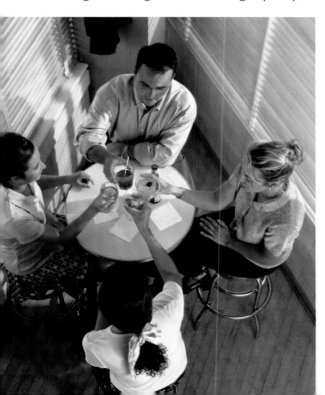

Self image and eating habits

The obvious reasons for selecting food are likes and dislikes, but they are only part of the process. Self-image can play a powerful role, one that leads to problems, particularly when matched by problems of self-confidence, concern or confusion about diet and external pressure to be something different. Weight, fitness and shape influence the way we feel about food. Being overweight and unfit may encourage destructive dieting, or comfort eating in an over-indulgent and negative sense. The worst scenario is that of yo-yo dieting and overeating.

Self-image also extends to the type of foods that are eaten and cooking practices. For example, while some men revel in the idea of being 'a bit of a chef', others would not dare admit to being kitchen competent. The cliché 'real men don't eat quiche' sums up a situation in which many 'macho' males will not even sample foods or dishes they consider to be too feminine – salads and yogurt are two examples – and it is alarming that many men still have this attitude.

Social taboos or image associations apply to women as well as men. Some women want to reassure the world that they are too hassled to cook, preferring to opt for pre-packed foods and ready meals as part of their image.

On a completely different level, a lack of interest in cooking and eating can be indicative of a lack of self-worth. This is not necessarily a social image association but a personal lack of self-value which may be linked to depression, or a milder 'feeling down' situation. This is particularly noticeable in those who have a history of eating well but who suddenly cannot be bothered, and it is often a real problem for those who live alone.

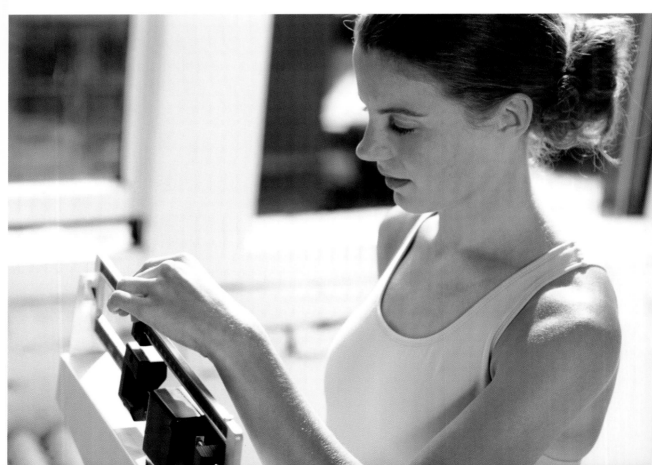

Dieting

The social pressure to be slim can be disastrous for many, especially young women – and, increasingly, men – who aim for an unrealistic body shape. Following a healthy, balanced eating plan and taking regular exercise is the best way of avoiding being overweight. Yo-yo dieting consisting of crash diets followed by over-indulgent periods of eating is not healthy – and it is just this type of approach to food that can be avoided when mind are body are in tune in terms of the food we choose to intake.

The urge to diet, and especially extreme dieting associated with eating disorders such as anorexia nervosa, often has other associations. A diet can be a call for help or attention, an expression of sadness or problems in areas other than eating, or a need to express the self-control which the person may feel they have lost in other areas of life. Indeed, the diet may not be a reflection of self-control but of the need to take control over other people or events. When a sensible diet is extended beyond the original target, associations should be assessed – is this diet for genuine, necessary weight loss or for other reasons? Are there rewards or positive feelings associated with the diet that should be translated into a new eating phase?

One of the best reasons any parent could have for finding the middle way with weight and diet is for the benefit of the next generation. It is sad to see children of pre-school age picking up parents' negative vibes about food. Little girls – and boys – often reflect the obsessions adults around them have about 'good' or 'bad' food, eating too much and being overweight. News reports frequently point out the problems that result.

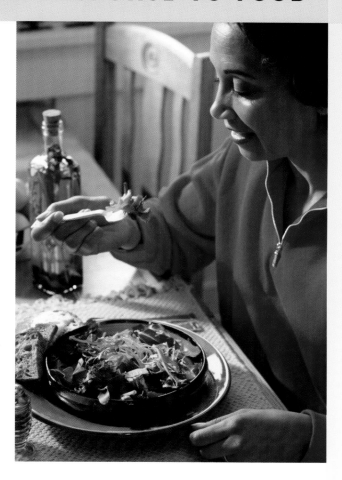

Anyone using a ladies' changing room at a sports club will have unavoidably overheard manic conversations about food, weight and appearance between women who clearly have diet problems and a poor attitude to food, and are unaware of the damage they are doing to their children playing nearby and listening.

Instead of using 'negative' dieting to overcome a poor mental state, adopting a really positive attitude to food and eating is far more successful. Focusing on self-appreciation and caring for the body may be the issue, then learning to eat the right foods for promoting a positive state of mind. Where weight loss is desirable, adopting a positive attitude to improving the body, aiming to be fitter and balancing the right nutrients is far preferable to sinking into a soul-destroying regime of counting calories.

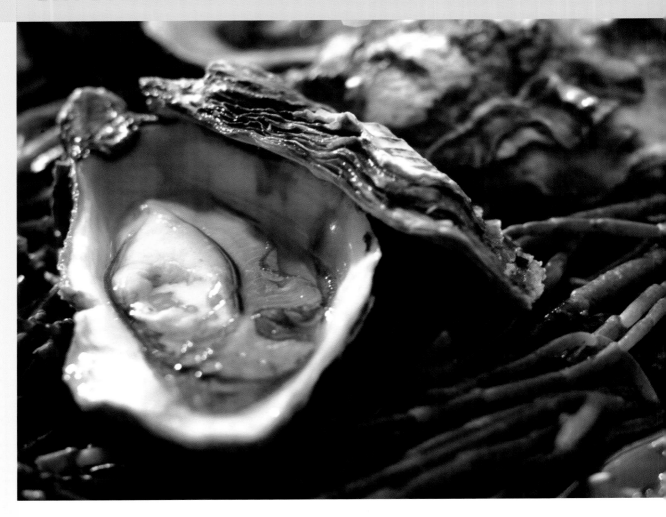

Food and sex

Freudian comparisons between the pleasures of feeding and sex are well known. Sigmund Freud, the Austrian physician known for the development of psychoanalysis and for his theories on the psychology of sex, linked the baby's first experience of sucking the mother's breast with sexual experiences later in life, suggesting that the instinct for sucking was the first basic sexual expression. He compared the baby's satisfaction of falling asleep after feeding with adult post-orgasmic bliss.

More general associations between food and sex stem from ancient theories and beliefs in the aphrodisiac powers of certain ingredients. General references to the aphrodisiac powers of food are not supported by evidence – even if the nutrients in some foods are important for the healthy functioning of the reproductive system, male or female. Most references to food aphrodisiacs are light-hearted, or used with reference to food in a sensual or romantic context. The perception of some foods and the ambience of dining can be linked with sex through taste, texture, appearance and the way, or circumstances, in which the food is eaten. Romantic or erotic, the link between food and sex is psychological rather than physiological.

Good food: positive eating

Nurturing a positive approach to food and eating is vital. You may not know exactly what you feel about food and eating. Ideas mingle and mix to create a collage of complex thoughts, or sometimes they become mixed and reduced to vague impressions. A simple way of sorting ideas about food is to make a split list, with positive thoughts on one side and negative on the other. If making the list in one session is too daunting, start the list on a notepad and add to it as you realise how you feel about food. Then read the list carefully with a view to exploring, resolving, counter-balancing and/or dispelling associations.

Reinforce the positive points by noting ways in which to build on them. For example, if one of the positive points is that you enjoy eating, reinforce this by listing all the good ingredients that you can cook and eat to promote a sense of wellbeing.

Cooking for your partner or family may be a positive point that also has negative associations, perhaps in terms of the time it takes or a lack of response from them. You may be able to reinforce the positive angle by looking at the types of dishes and foods you cook or by introducing them to the idea of cooking with you, so that you pass on your knowledge and share the pleasure.

If you enjoy eating home-cooked food as a positive point but on a negative level find it time consuming, then reinforce the positive by thinking of the preparation or cooking stage as a means of therapeutic relaxation

Negative ideas may including time-consuming shopping and the answer could be to re-schedule the shopping or to make the best

use of freezer and fridge for keeping ample food supplies in the house. Instead of lumping all the shopping together into one mammoth supermarket trawl, making several short trips for a few items can be less stressful and more convenient. Being too ambitious can lead to negative thoughts on cooking, with failures, mess or exhaustion as a result; the answer is to focus on one or two simple dishes or cooking methods and build on these as your confidence increases.

If you eat a lot of convenience foods, you may find home-made dishes bland by comparison – this could be due to the high levels of salt, sugar, fat and flavourings in the dishes you buy. As you change your diet you will begin to appreciate the lighter, natural flavour of ingredients and discover that they are full of nuances completely lost in the over-seasoned, ready-made commercial products.

If you have several unresolved negative items, look through the pages that follow for support and solutions. Keep your original list and reassess it as you embark on a new approach to food. You may be happily surprised at the shift towards the positive.

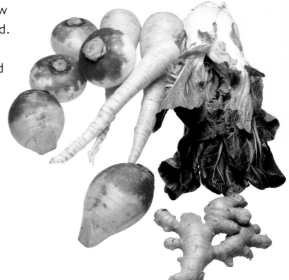

NATURAL INSTINCTS: CARING & SHARING

While the anticipation of eating and enjoying a meal may naturally provide pleasure, the process of planning, shopping and cooking is also innately satisfying. Demanding Western lifestyles leave little room for simple pleasures, and sophisticated solutions replace basics in too many instances. From necessity, the majority of planning and shopping tasks have been streamlined, and cosmopolitan convenience foods have replaced the simplest quick dishes. When we think about whether we are delighted with the way things are, we realise that streamlining and de-humanizing takes the heart out of eating. If food and eating is no longer personal to you and your family or friends, if it has become a necessity to which you are only distantly connected, pause to find the soul in food and look for the spirit of good eating.

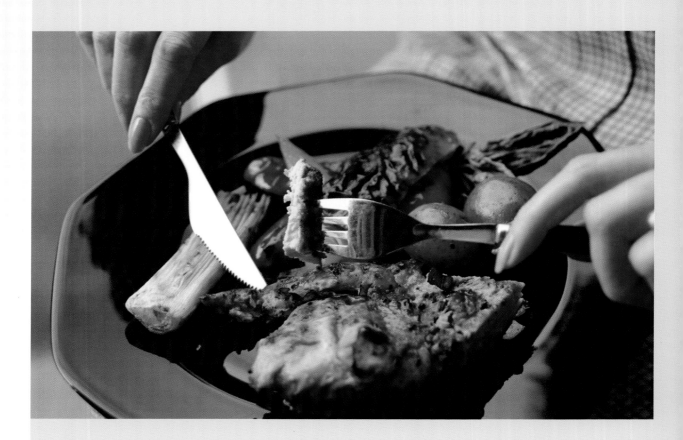

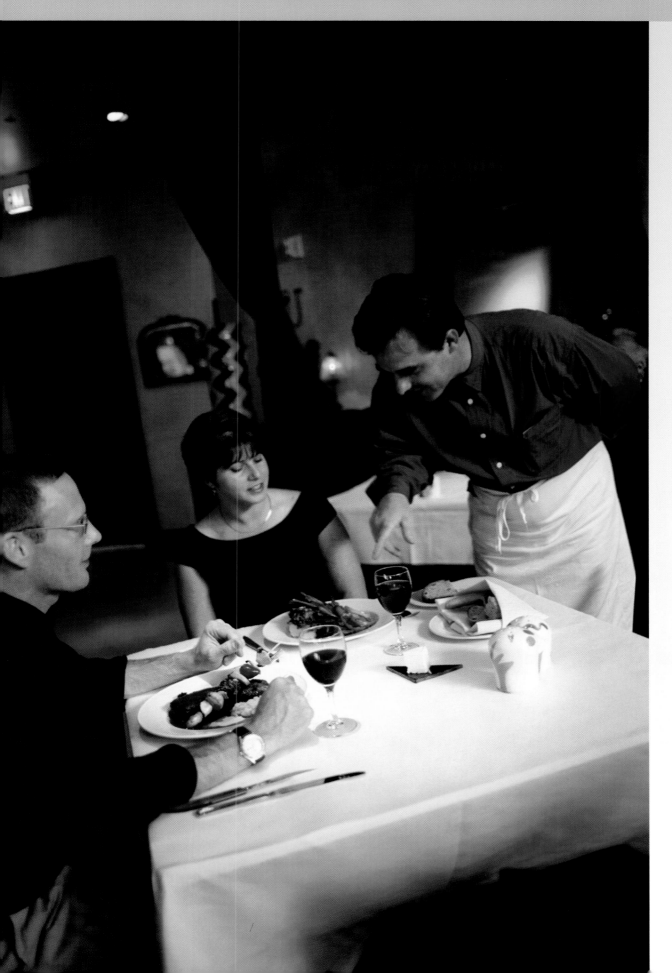

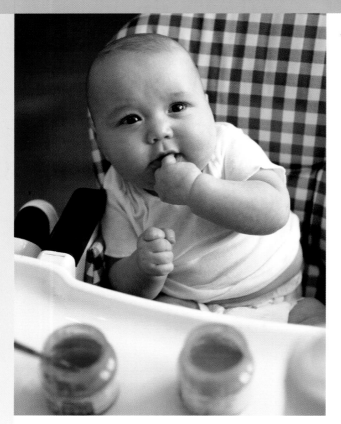

Introduction to food: feeding and weaning

We are born with the need to feed, and seeking out the mother's breast is one of the first instincts in life. From the parent's viewpoint, feeding is one of the fundamental aspects of caring for a baby, developing into weaning and teaching the child to feed itself.

The first introduction to food encompasses a whole range of practices and emotions for the parent as well as for the child. The need to care for and nurture the infant is part of the sense of responsibility. It is not just a case of giving milk or food but of ensuring that the child is learning to take in enough milk and developing a hunger for, and ability to eat, the right food during weaning.

Everyone emphasizes the need for a positive approach during those first introductions to food. Feeding is more than a mechanical activity of imparting nourishment, requiring patient, loving and encouraging attention. It is also one of the first sources of interaction between the parent and child, and one of the first teaching processes.

Providing for others

Cooking for and feeding the young child continues to be a focus for caring. The vital emphasis on nutrition is matched by loving encouragement and coaxing. Teaching a child to eat imparts social skills, once the basic mechanics of getting food to mouth can be achieved.

The aura of caring extends well beyond the minutes or hours spent on feeding. Selecting the right foods, preparing and heating or cooking them are all part of the feeding process. Teaching the child how to approach and eat food, overcoming rejection and introducing the idea of food choices are important; then there is the notion of sharing the eating experience (rather than mimicry) and the process of deciding on what to eat or cook, as well as preparing the food.

Caring for the nourishment of babies and children is essential, and extending this to others can be a way of bonding with them and displaying affection. In the majority of households the woman is most likely to be the person to organize food and meals for the family. Much of the concern and attention that is paid to this is unconscious, some of it a matter of routine but usually with additional care. Cooking for friends, or sharing food with them, is a similar way of expressing affection, often in a different, more conscious, way than preparing routine family meals.

Cooking Together

Make time to enjoy cooking occasionally. It is such a beneficial activity that it is good to share it with other members of the family.

• Plan simple cooking sessions with your children. Make fun, good foods and try to cover a range of recipes on different occasions. For example, try biscuits, little cakes, a tasty dip with crunchy vegetable sticks or a fruit pudding.

• Involve your partner in cooking, from planning a special meal that can be extremely simple, through shopping for the ingredients and enjoying the experience of cooking together. If culinary adventures are not your forte, do not try to be too ambitious – the exercise is not to stretch skills but to discover the caring side of cooking. It could be no more than the preparation of tea and toast or making sandwiches together.

• Involve the whole household in meal preparation in a positive way. Try to bring the family together on one occasion a week when everyone can share something of the preparation before sitting down together. The food does not have to be elaborate but the meal should include a contribution from everyone, from laying the table to helping with stirring or mixing, tasting or seasoning a dish.

• Share cooking sessions with friends, making them informal and fun.

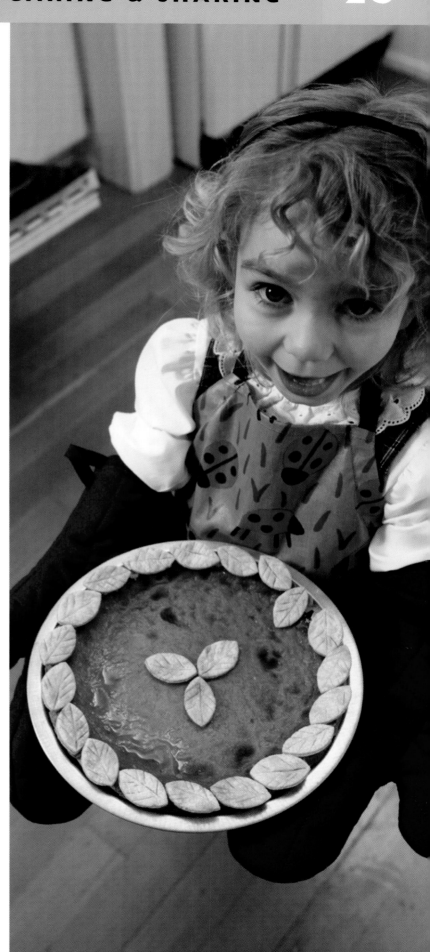

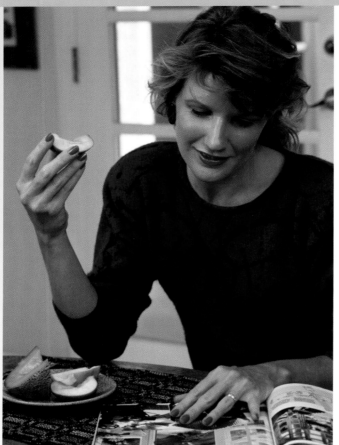

The idea of shopping and cooking for one may seem selfish or self-indulgent, or too much effort, but we all have a responsibility to ourselves. This extends beyond eating a balanced diet to achieving all the benefits of focusing on mealtimes and dining situations. When you live alone, it is all too easy to grab a quick snack or dismiss the idea of a good ambience for eating; it is also easy to get out of the habit of entertaining and sharing meals at home with friends. Yet these are all the positive associations with shopping, food and cooking that make us feel so much better about ourselves and others.

Providing for yourself

One of the important aspects of caring for children and youngsters is making sure that, as they grow up, they learn how to look after themselves. Anyone living alone has to shop, cook and eat, and today's society has an increasing number of people who live alone. Although many happily live alone from choice, others have circumstances forced upon them – bereaved of partners or unwillingly single through separation, they find themselves in negative situations. Adopting a self-caring attitude to eating alone is not always easy, especially for those who may be depressed or lacking self-esteem. Taking positive control of eating for wellbeing is equally difficult for those leading a frenetic single lifestyle that is overfilled with work or packed with away-from-home activities.

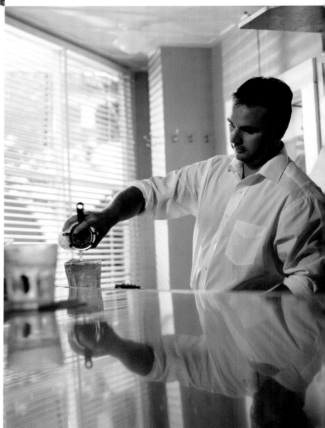

Wellbeing for one

Thinking about practical ways to make the most of food and cooking work is a good starting point for reviving a dull approach to eating.

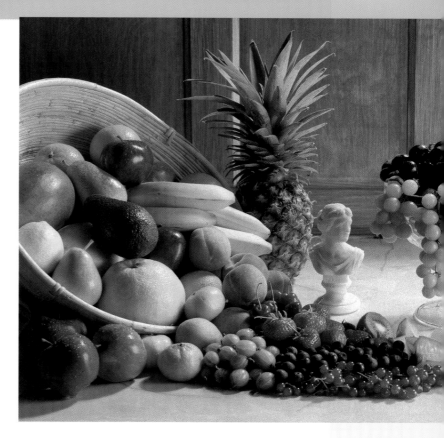

- Review your diet by making lists of what you eat and what you would like to, or think you should, eat. Do not think of this in a silly or indulgent sense but in a balanced, 'good for me' sense. Write down all the dishes, products and ingredients you eat (no need for a meal order as long as it is all there). Then list the foods and dishes you would enjoy in an ideal world – at a restaurant or when eating with friends. What about foods you would like in a good and balanced diet? How do the lists compare? If the reality falls far short of the ideal, how can you introducing desirable foods? Now go for the 'get-real' list for putting the spirit back into your diet. For example, include main ingredients you select from restaurant menus, or make some of those salads that sound so stylish and are, in fact, incredibly simple. Include some super-foods and dishes – brilliant breakfast muesli, fabulous fruit drinks or a glorious fresh fruit salad.

- Make some time for calm food shopping. It does not have to be a regular event but it is a good idea when assembling a modest 'storecupboard' of positive ingredients, including frozen foods. For example, allow time to look through all the freezers in the supermarket and select some of the excellent vegetables; buy a few cans of beans and pulses, salmon or anchovies; look for fresh pasta (it will freeze well); and check out the dried pasta and grains, such as couscous, rice or bulghur.

- Think about foods that you enjoy preparing and/or dishes you like to cook, and allow sufficient time for it to be relaxing.

- Plan a few special meals for yourself. Make them special in the rounded sense of including good ingredients – look through the recipe chapters and select dishes that really appeal to you.

- Make the effort to serve the food well, on attractive dishes, laid on a table or stylishly on a tray.

- Allow time to sit and enjoy some proper meals, rather than relying too often on the grab-a-snack approach.

- Aim for a positive ambience when eating. If you enjoy eating in front of the television, be selective about the type of programme rather than collapsing in front of anything. Try listening to the radio or music instead.

Stocking up - security and satisfaction

Before freezer space became essential, convenience foods and the onset of 24 hour shopping, the 'housewife' was said to gain immense satisfaction from shopping and stocking up. She was viewed as a squirrel figure, stacking away her cans of salmon and peas, and home-cooked preserves to her own immense sense of achievement and for the benefit of the family around whom she centred her life. While the whole image is anathema to the majority of today's women, there is truth in the feeling of security and satisfaction that can be derived from shopping and storing food.

Shopping therapy is recognized in the supermarket environment as well as that of clothes and leisure goods. There are two

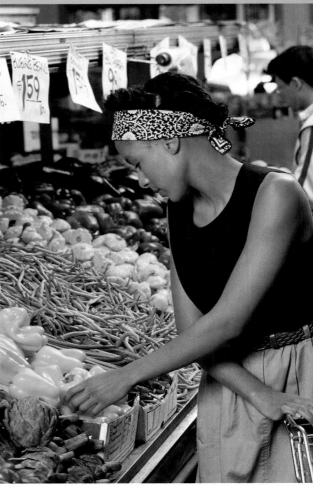

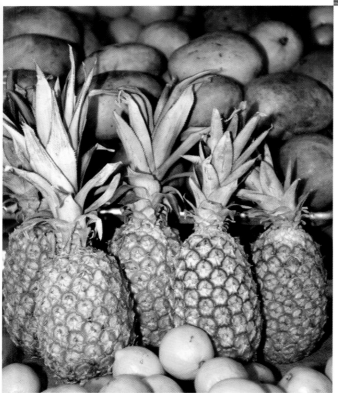

types of foods shopping – the essential, stocking up on basics kind, and the non-essential, luxury or indulgent items for which we browse when time allows. Good feelings from shopping also stem from being organized and focusing in advance on selecting foods that are healthy. Buying lots of fresh fruit and vegetables, attractive breads and storecupboard ingredients that help with healthy eating results in a warm, virtuous glow as the shopping trolley is wheeled away.

Fitting in food

If food and eating is so basic, why should anyone be so concerned about its value other than as a source of nourishment? In the 'fifties and 'sixties Abraham Maslow, an American psychologist, explored ideas about our relative needs and associated personality in terms of self-fulfilment – or, to use his term, self-actualization .

His theories are often represented as a pyramid of needs, with basic physiological needs at the bottom, followed by safety, belonging, esteem and self-actualization.

Maslow suggested that each stage of the pyramid had to be achieved before an individual – or a society – could move on to the next, and that some would not progress to the top. Fairly obviously, the basic survival needs, including water and food, are at the bottom of the triangle. Above this, there is a need for security and protection, followed by a desire for social belonging, affection and love. Self-esteem and ego, along with dignity and achieving the respect of others, comes next. At the top of the pyramid, when all other layers are satisfied to the individual's requirements, there is the possibility for achieving self-actualization or fulfilment, in whatever form that may be. Within the context of society and/or lifestyle, the stages of our needs apply in relative value.

In sophisticated Western society, where the basic physiological needs are met and taken for granted, the role of food consumerism fits into the higher levels of the pyramid. Cooking and eating are important for expressing and receiving love in a caring and sharing sense, and to maintain self-esteem. The type of foods we eat, in terms of the whole business of belonging, is also important.

self-actualization

esteem, self-respect, approval

belonging, affection, friendship, love

safety, security, protection

physiological needs, air, water, food

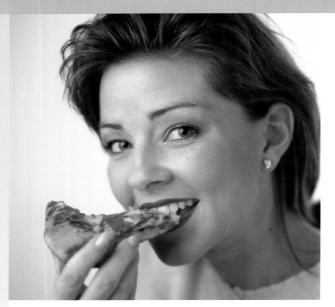

Food etiquette and meal occasions

Teaching children about eating also involves etiquette and table manners, which vary widely. Beyond a basic standard, the majority of people practise various levels of food etiquette according to the occasion. For example, relaxing in front of the television with a bowl of pasta for supper does not call for the same behaviour as a formal dinner party. The ambience and interaction are quite different in each case; and the personal perception and satisfaction are not the same.

To share positive eating experiences there must be a certain mutual respect for mealtime manners. Collapsing in a chair with a snack in front of the television does not allow time for interacting with others over a meal. Sitting around a table as a family, a couple, or with friends is more sociable. Family meals around the table are often criticized as occasions for controversy and argument, especially with a teenage family, but they are also constructive occasions for airing opinions, finding areas of mutual agreement and, in a media-dominated world, talking. The more frequent, or at least regular, the meals, the more likely they are to be harmonious and beneficial.

Between couples, and with friends or relations, establishing a routine or, at least, occasions for sharing meals in a relaxed, sociable atmosphere is excellent for nurturing respect and enjoyment. The comparatively minor constraints of sitting down to a formal meal can suddenly make people regard each other as individuals and as people in their own right. For many couples, a meal together provides a pause from a busy schedule. Remembering to take time out for sharing meals is a good ethos in a fraught lifestyle.

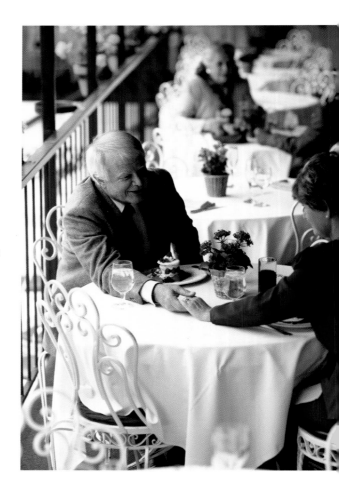

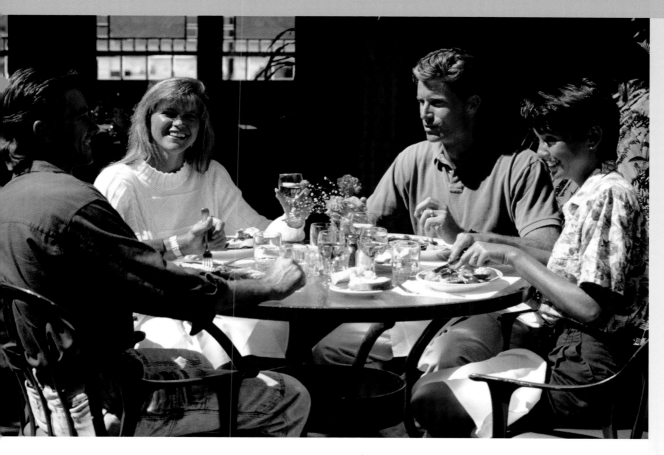

Meals together

Planning enjoyable eating occasions is not difficult and a change from the norm can be enough. Looking for interaction and a caring ambience is a simple aim.

- Quite simply, eat together as a household.

- Prepare a table or breakfast area in the kitchen, making a neat and appealing place to eat.

- If you normally eat at a table in a dull or negative atmosphere, try to change this by moving the table, rearranging the usual seating or making the table setting more attractive than usual. Try different lighting or unobtrusive background music.

- Eating a completely different type of dish is a good way to make a relaxing change. Dishes that are shared are ideal, such as fondue.

- Instead of serving out food onto plates in the kitchen, take serving dishes to the table so that everyone can help themselves. This encourages social interaction and a greater appreciation of the food, all of which makes eating more enjoyable.

- In warm weather, try eating outdoors to promote a different, positive atmosphere.

- A picnic or packed lunch can be a good opportunity for enjoying eating together.

FOOD & FORM: COOKING STYLES & METHODS

The appearance of food almost always arouses a response. Why are the fresh fruit and vegetables displayed in the most inconvenient place in the supermarket in terms of loading a shopping trolley? Probably because they look fresh, clean and inviting as you walk in through the door. It is certainly not logical in terms of where they should be in the trolley. Shuffling around tender tomatoes and easily bruised, leafy vegetables as heavy bags of flour, cans, bottles and laundry products are added makes no sense at all – yet that is what we do because the retailer wants us to feel good about the supermarket when we first walk in. Coming straight up against a stack of toilet rolls is not the same as facing an array of colourful fruit and vegetables as you walk in through the door.

The colours, shapes, aroma and healthy image of the fresh produce makes us feel good. It has an invigorating influence, especially as this is an area where we can handle and feel the food, discovering the textures and becoming directly involved with it. This reaction to food is just one of many, and nurturing such good associations with our essential nourishment can be life-enhancing.

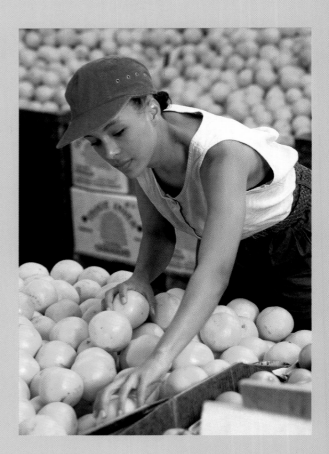

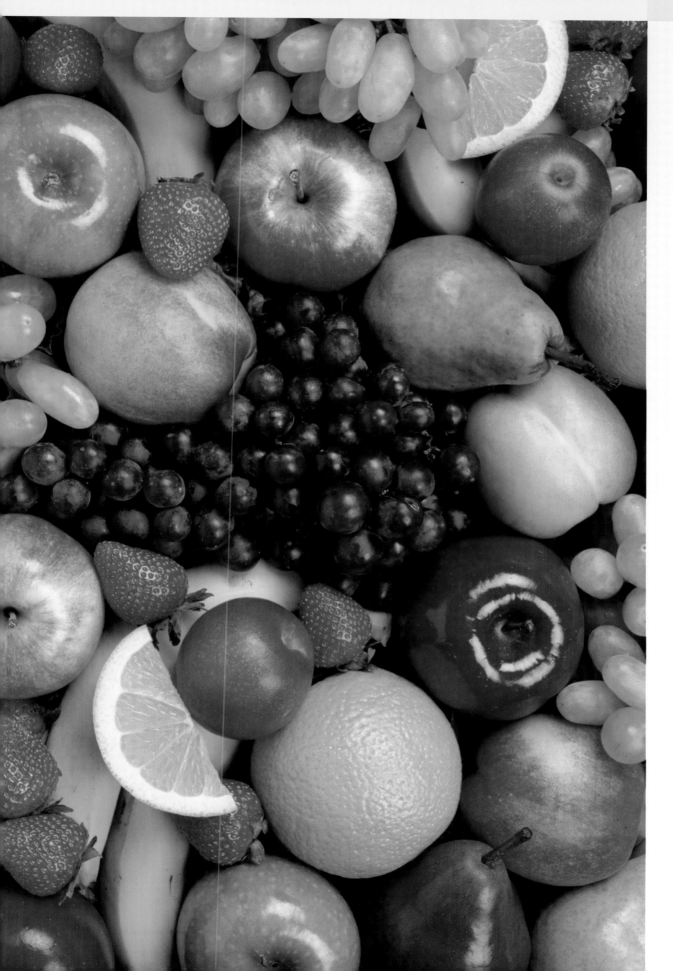

Hunger and appetite

What makes us hungry? Our bodies let us know when we need water and food by thirst and hunger. When the stomach is empty and energy supplies fall, we become hungry. So how come we do not have the same urge to stop eating when the body has taken in sufficient food? The physical mechanisms for letting us know that we have eaten enough to provide the body with all it needs are not efficient. Feeling full is a relative sensation and it takes time for food to be digested, so, unlike the lack of energy that promotes hunger, there is no 'energy stores replenished' indicator for us to rely on.

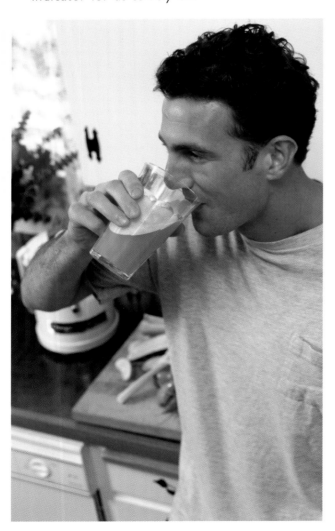

In addition to the physical indicators, appetite is a sensation influenced by a variety and mix of other factors. These include habit, environment and situation, mood or state of mind, the appearance of food, and the smell, taste, flavour and texture of food.

Eating habits

We grow used to eating at certain times. When we eat regular meals, our bodies expect food and we feel hungry in anticipation. When we alter our meal patterns, our bodies get used to new routines over a number of days as, for example, when work-day routines change during holidays. Getting back to eating a lunchtime sandwich after relaxing over a substantial holiday lunch is always tedious. We also may find that eating early in the evening instead of later is a hard holiday habit to break.

Eating habits – meal times and the type of foods or dishes eaten – can provoke good or bad feelings, or indeed nothing other than a sense of routine. That routine can give a feeling of security, especially to children, the elderly or anyone who may depend on meals as a main point of reference in the day. The fact that we are able to change eating habits means that we can alter the influence they have on our lives. This means that we can adjust what we eat, and when and how we eat it, to maximize the enjoyment, relaxation or other benefits from food.

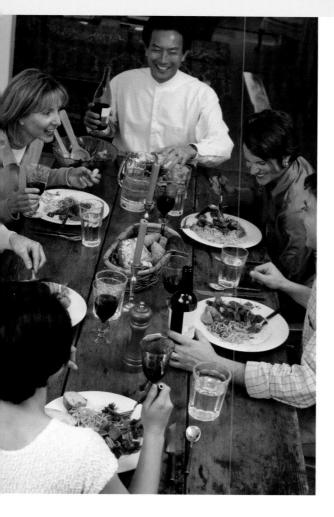

Environment and circumstances

Have you ever gone out for a meal in a fairly undecided frame of appetite only to become quite hungry as soon as you look at the menu outside the restaurant door? Environment and circumstances promote appetite even when we do not necessarily feel hunger. Both factors also influence our response to the hunger and eating situation – going out for a meal is usually a pleasant experience and the whole eating situation makes us feel good. Conversely, rushing around a supermarket or coping with stressful environments can work up an appetite, either immediately or shortly afterwards. The idea of eating can be as a source of comfort.

This is another aspect we can control to help us feel good. Instead of allowing food to be a desperate antidote to a stressful situation, a meal can be planned to pre-empt the problem. An energy-giving, healthy snack, or a relaxing light meal can be excellent alternatives to impromptu comfort snacking on chocolate and sweets or high-fat savoury snack products.

- Plan some regular meal occasions that allow time to relax and enjoy eating. Ideally, schedule in some space in which to enjoy the preparation of the food.

- Within busy family schedules, plan regular, if occasional, meals for the entire household to share. Allow for flexibility, but do not give up on the idea of sharing family meals as a matter of habit. Let family meals, or shared meals as a couple, become a point for social refuelling and a positive sharing of minds and spirits.

- Allow regular spaces for important meals or snacks that leave you, as an individual, feeling mentally replenished.

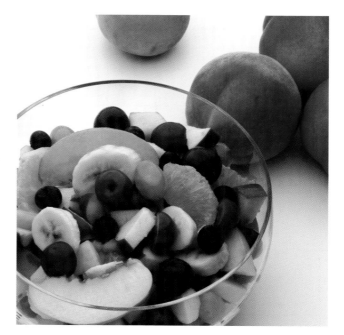

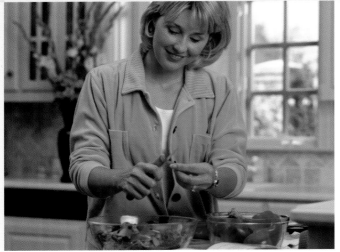

Appearance of food

Being presented with or looking at appetizing food makes us want to eat. The look of different foods promotes various feelings – just as a vibrant display of fruit and vegetables is uplifting, an array of breads may be calming, or a steaming-hot chocolate pudding may appear comforting.

Mood or state of mind

This needs no introduction as an appetite stimulant. All sorts of moods make us feel hungry – when we celebrate we do so by eating a special meal; if we are sad we take comfort in the reassurance of food; if we feel worried, we seek solace in the safety of having food to eat; when boredom strikes, eating is the perfect distraction; and when we want to relax we are likely to plan a gentle meal. Instead of allowing mood to unexpectedly dictate appetite, reverse the situation and make the most of food and eating to promote a positive state of mind.

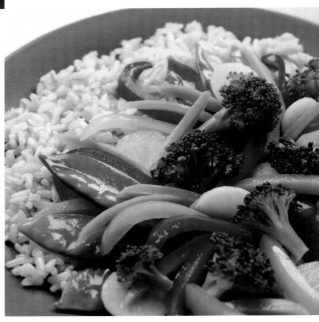

- Be aware of mental needs and plan meals accordingly. For example, focus on meals that promote calm when situations are likely to be stressful, or include plenty of foods for a sense of vitality during energetic periods.

- Cooking therapy can be an excellent opportunity to relax or re-vitalize, especially when preparing meals to help promote a positive state of mind.

- Be aware of diet as a source of assistance in overcoming mood swings, for example those associated with pre-menstrual tension.

When shopping, or cooking and sitting down to eat a meal, the ingredients, cooking methods and dishes all influence the state of mind. This is especially true in the sense that handling and preparing some colourful and lively looking ingredients will lift the spirits. Some cooking methods, as well as the texture and appearance of the food as it is being prepared, can be quite therapeutic.

Aroma, texture and flavour

The aroma, texture and flavour of ingredients and dishes work together to influence the whole sensation of taste. Individually, these characteristics can exert great influence over appetite, our pre-consumption appreciation of food, the sense of anticipation and, ultimately, our mood and attitude.

This is true at every point of interaction with food, from walking into a specialist delicatessen and experiencing the heady aromas or being surrounded by the shapes, forms and textures of the ingredients to feeling and smelling ingredients as we cut and combine them, then finally to experiencing the finished dish before, during and after eating it. And the follow-on sensations associated with food are important. The impressions, memories or lingering sense of wellbeing can help to maintain the good that positive food associations bring.

While this seems personal, and it is easy to make the most of positive food aspects as an individual, sharing these food sentiments with others is easy. Every time we cook for, or eat with, others, we share our food likes and dislikes, passing on our impressions in more than spoken terms with our body language and enthusiasm.

The texture of food influences the way in which it can be eaten and the ambience of the dining situation. Moist and liquid foods have been associated with sensual experiences and it has been suggested that preparing them for others is an expression of particular care or affection; within a sexual context the moist foods are considered to be more suggestive of love and allure. There is certainly some connection between warming drinks and soups and a sense of caring, while cool and crisp foods are less personal and invigorating. The associations could be as much to do with the manner in which we eat these foods as the food itself.

Dry foods, on the other hand, have been associated with less caring and, in the sexual sense, indicative of a lack of attraction. However, as with the majority of associations between food and sex, this has to be taken with a pinch of salt, so to speak, as the shape of what we eat is thought of as being equally important. Asparagus spears and the way they are (correctly) eaten with the fingers, dripping with melted butter, are considered to be among the most sexy of foods – and although they are dry, there is all that melted butter.

Cooking methods

Levi-Strauss, a French anthropologist, in looking at the influence of nature or culture on the placing of raw or cooked food in the pattern of human cooking methods, suggested that roasting was a basic cooking method, close to nature for its associations with fire. Boiling was a method exposed to culture for its use of a pot and the technique of cooking in water. Grilling (broiling) came closest to the eating of raw food, steaming was between roasting and boiling, and frying was closer to cultural influences for its use of oil. Patterns of cooking methods and the associations they have with our natural or cultured sense is not immediately relevant to the idea of food therapy and promoting a sense of wellbeing. However, it supports the idea of an association between food and the practical and innate aspects of the human character.

Some food preparation is gentle, steady or repetitive and it can be calming, soothing or reassuring. Repeated cutting, as when slicing or dicing, comes into this category. Gentle stirring and mixing is also calming or soothing. Kneading can be reassuring, calming and comforting, although it can also be a way to relieve frustrations and express anger. This, in the context of finding positive links with food and its preparation, is not to be encouraged. (It is a good idea to avoid linking any negative feelings with food.)

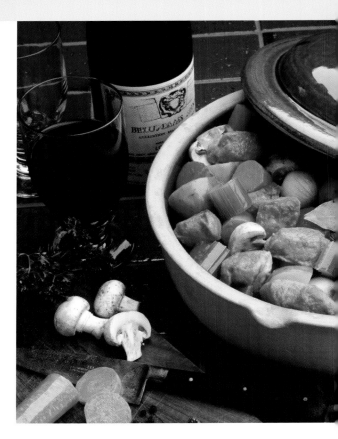

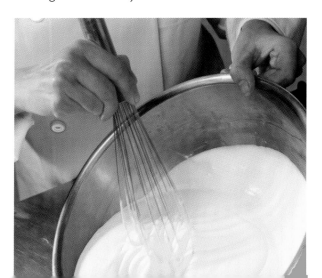

Slow braising, stewing and simmering are gentle, calming methods. The food can often be left to continue cooking unattended. The aromas they impart are gentle or background by nature, or rich and reassuring. Baking brings a mixture of messages, from calming or energetic in the preparation to complex measuring and mixing that can be incredibly absorbing and satisfying. The cooking process brings heartwarming smells and reassurance, along with a very particular sense of encouragement and energy.

Lively stir-frying is vigorous and vital, and an excellent method for bringing life to food preparation and meals. The resulting ingredients and dishes are full of textures, intermingling flavours and energy. Sautéing (correctly carried out this is a slightly tamer version of stir-frying done in a frying pan, turning and rearranging the food all the time) and frying are also fast and bright methods. Grilling and roasting are not as energetic, but they involve high-heat and are generally enlivening.

Kitchen equipment

Take a new look at old equipment to revamp your attitude to food. For a positive approach be brutal with bashed-up pans, tatty and chipped bowls and containers, and knives that have lost their edge. Discard dust collectors and throw out items that are well past their best. Revitalize your attitude with carefully selected tools that you will use, building up a limited number of items as you need them.

It is so easy to accumulate all sorts of crockery and cutlery that gradually becomes sad and unappealing. Sometimes we just outgrow items, especially those that were fashion whims, and they serve only as reminders of the past rather than as positive

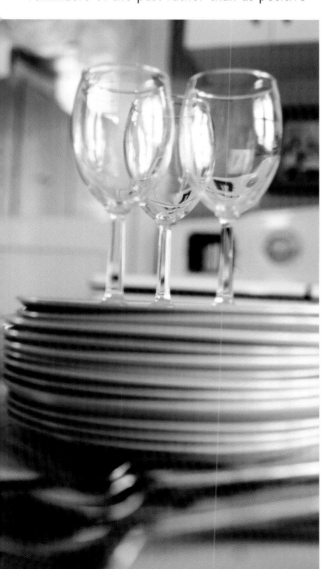

icons for the future. There is nothing better for encouraging a new interest in eating than a simple collection of inexpensive everyday dishes off which to serve and eat. Clean lines, simple colours – if any, plain white is usually best – and sturdy but not clumsy design works wonders for most foods and provides diners with a sense of satisfaction and reassurance. Rely on accessories and asides for adding fun and vitality – table napkins and inexpensive glassware, and a selection of different cups or mugs are practical. And taking the trouble to use accessories, such as table napkins, is a positive step in recognizing the value of eating.

Sort out storecupboards and check the range of foods you keep in stock. It is better to have a modest supply of good condiments, seasonings and ingredients than a vast stock that is rarely used, diminished in flavour and quality and serving only to confuse the choice when you want to make decisions on what to cook.

Once the kitchen's excess has been shed, keep requirements in focus to prevent a build-up of unwanted clutter. Clutter serves only to make cooking and eating unnecessarily difficult and complicated. Simplicity assists with the search for the soul in cooking and eating.

GOOD FOOD:

ESSENTIAL EATING

*A*chieving a balanced diet does more than simply help to ensure good physical health – it really does bring a positive attitude to life. This section briefly outlines the main functions of the different types of food in the physical sense by looking at the various food groups. Then it moves on to focus on the types of foods that are likely to promote good mental development and a general sense of wellbeing.

The aim is to find harmony in food and eating. Once you are familiar with the physical needs – the types of food that bring the right nutrients in the correct proportions – then you can concentrate on enjoying food and cooking. Recognise the innate pleasure in eating with which we are all endowed and build on this in a positive sense to find the spirit in cooking – or even create your own!

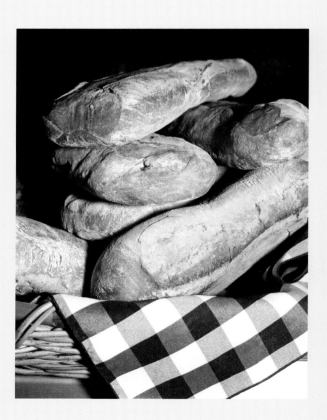

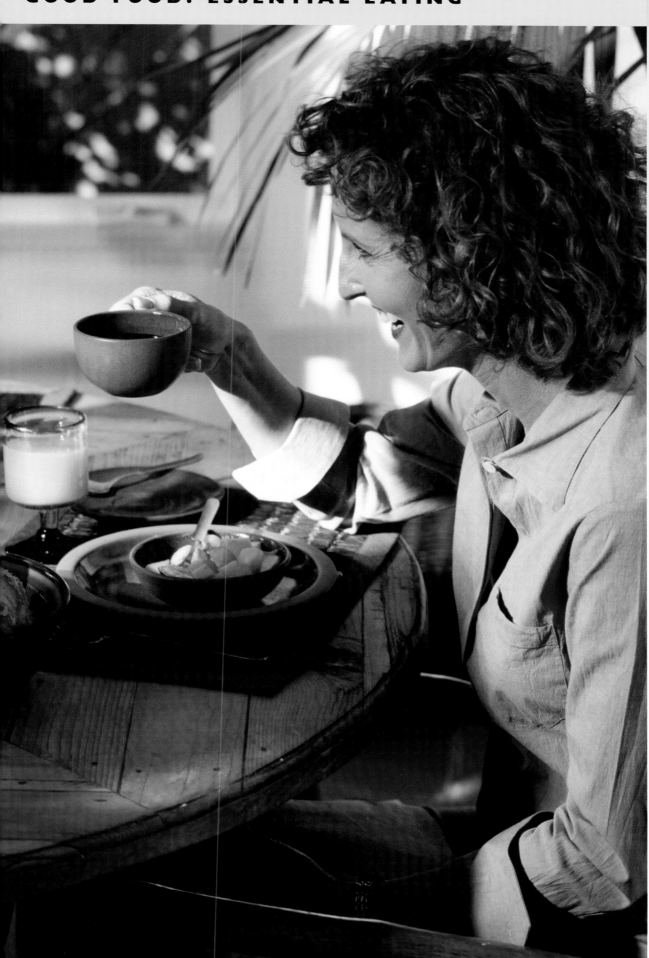

A personal attitude to eating

Diet is personal and requirements vary according to lifestyle and metabolism. Maintaining a healthy weight is a fundamental requirement that depends on balancing diet with energy used – but this does not mean trying to achieve a ridiculously low weight or model figure. On the contrary, it is most important to find your own healthy, active weight and endeavour to maintain it. The best starting point for this may well be a visit to your doctor.

There are no such things as unhealthy foods, but some items can be eaten in unhealthy quantities. Variety and balance are the important features in an enjoyable, long-term diet. Eating lots of different types of food provides a good range of nutrients.

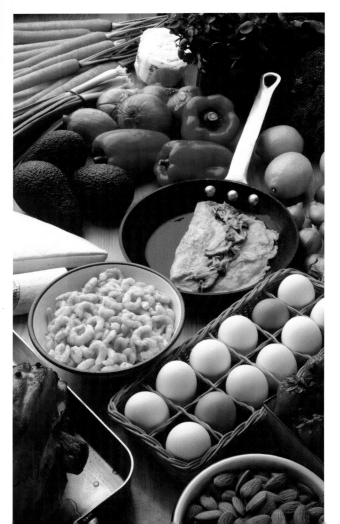

Balancing a diet means eating different types of food in the proportions the body needs them. The general recommendation is to include plenty of plant foods and ample supplies of starch, a good fibre content, modest amounts of low-fat protein, oily fish and a little fat. The other basic requirement is to eat more or less the right amount of food in relation to the energy expended to avoid becoming unhealthily overweight.

- Starchy carbohydrates like bread, potatoes, pasta, rice and other grains – provide the best source of energy. They are satisfying and the right type of food to fill up on.

- Fruit and vegetables are vital for vitamins and minerals as well as other benefits, and they should be eaten in generous quantities. Health experts recommend that five portions of fruit and vegetables should be eaten daily. Plant foods in particular play a valuable protective role. The importance of vitamins, minerals and fibre is well established; the extent of the contribution from other components in plant foods is only just being discovered.

- Proteins are essential for growth and repair of the body, but they are not needed in as large a proportion as vegetables and starches. Animal sources of protein – including fish, poultry and meat – should be balanced by vegetable proteins, such as beans and pulses.

- Fats are important in the diet, but only in modest proportions, so foods that are high in fat should not be eaten regularly in large quantities. Animal fats, in particular, should be limited.

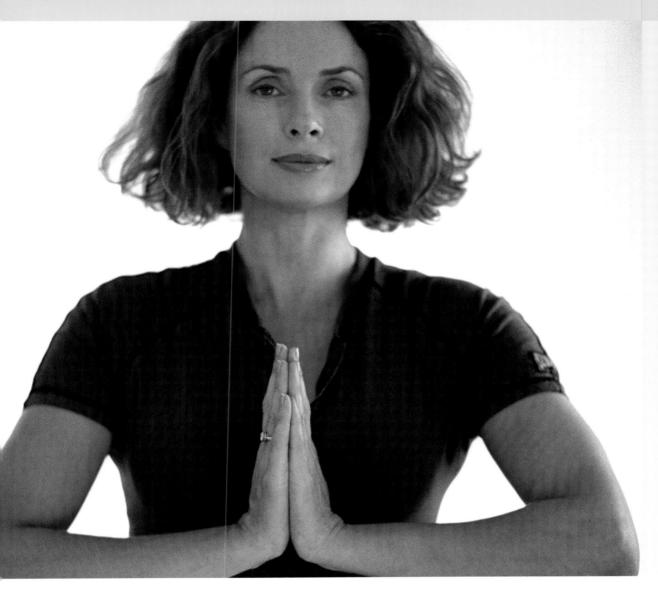

Exercise and relaxation

Exercise and relaxation work in tandem, to the benefit of mind and body. While exercise promotes physical fitness, it can also be a most effective means of working out negative energy – the frustrations, fears and inadequacies suffered in everyday life. The importance of consulting a doctor before embarking on any exercise programme for the first time, or after a period of comparative inactivity, must be stressed. Exercise should not be over-demanding or viewed as a chore, but it should be selected for enjoyment and balance so that it is energizing; it should not become obsessive. The right level and type of exercise should act as a means of relaxation.

There is also a need for quiet, calm and personal relaxation. This may be as simple as dedicated stretching following exercise, or a simple process of unwinding at key moments in the day or, at least, at the end of the day, before going to bed. There are many options and the choice is personal: all it has to be is something that works for you. Relaxation is especially important for a good sleep pattern.

A Guide to Nutrients

The functions of separate nutrients may be different, but they work closely together to keep the body machine running smoothly.

Carbohydrates are starches (complex carbohydrates) and sugars (simple carbohydrates). They are the satisfying foods and the providers of energy. Starchy foods should form the base for a healthy diet. Energy is released slowly from complex carbohydrates, so not only do they feel filling when first eaten but they also provide a steady source of energy for some time.

It is important to eat starches that are unrefined and high in fibre, as well as the more refined types. For example, some wholemeal bread should be included as well as white bread. Breakfast cereals and whole grains are also valuable.

Fibre is carbohydrate that the body cannot digest and break down completely, so it is passed out of the body. Fibre absorbs liquid to provide bulk and moisture for the waste products of digestion, allowing them to be excreted easily and preventing constipation. There are different types of fibre, some from fruit and vegetables and others from starchy carbohydrates. A good mixture of different types, including soluble fibre from oats and the pectin content of fruit, is helpful for moderating cholesterol levels in the body.

Sugars occur naturally in some vegetables and many fruits, and these naturally sweet foods can make good sweeteners instead of using pure sugar. There is nothing wrong with sugar but it can be eaten to excess as it provides 'empty' calories. Eating lots of sugary snacks and sweet foods can result in a weight problem. High-sugar snacks and sweet, acidic drinks cause dental caries, particularly in children and young people. There is nothing wrong with sweets as an occasional treat, but not as a regular part of the diet.

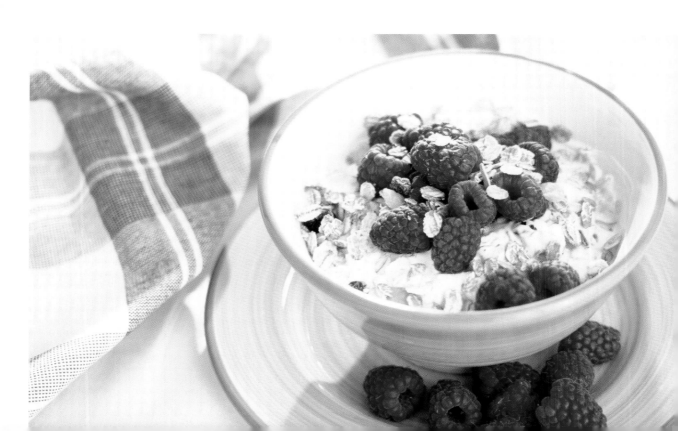

Protein

Fish, poultry and meat are the main animal protein foods. Dairy produce, such as eggs, cheese and milk, is also a source. Proteins are made up of amino acids, eight of which are essential and they are all provided in animal protein. Plant sources of protein do not include all the essential amino acids in any one food, with the exception of soya beans, which are a source of high-quality protein. Other beans and pulses, rice and grains provide protein. When a good mix of vegetable foods is eaten the body obtains all the amino acids it needs.

Fat

Fatty acids are essential in the diet. Fats are known as saturated or unsaturated: the unsaturated fats may be polyunsaturated or mono-unsaturated. Animal fats tend to have a higher content of saturated fat than vegetable fats. The amount of the fat in the diet should be limited to a small amount daily and the majority of the fat we eat should be unsaturated. High-fat foods, such as butter, cheese, cream, fatty meats, oils and oil-based spreads and dressings, should be used in modest amounts. Oily fish should be eaten regularly – ideally twice a week – to provide the valuable omega-3 fatty acids

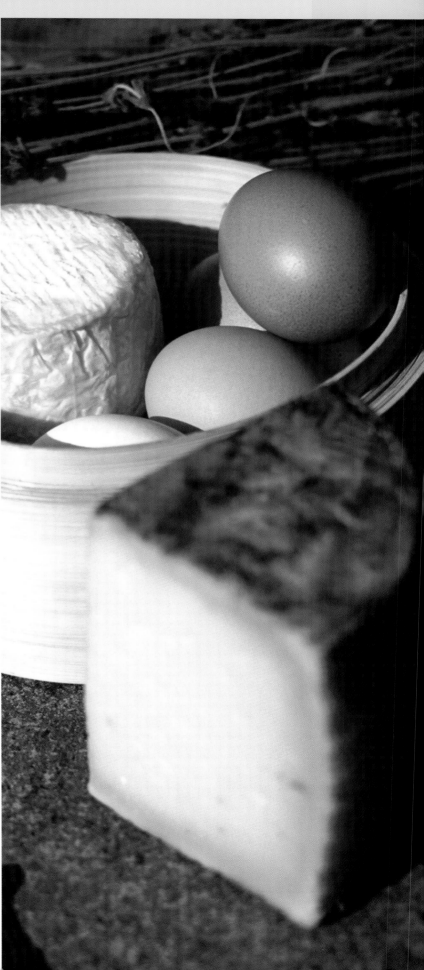

Vitamins

Vitamins are found in a wide variety of foods and they fulfil many general or specific functions. These are the catalysts that spark off essential bodily processes or ensure that they work successfully. They also help to protect the body against infection, disease and damage, and maintain general good health. Vitamins are grouped into water-soluble types – vitamins C and B group – and fat-soluble types – vitamins A, D, E and K.

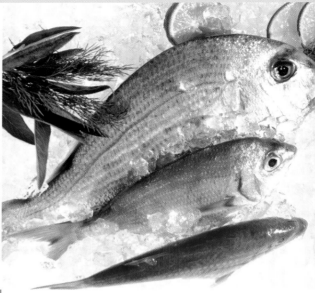

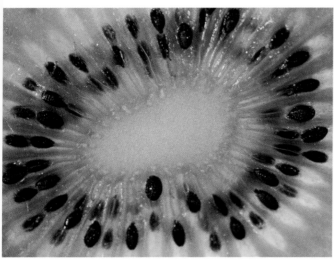

Water-Soluble Vitamins

The body does not store water-soluble vitamins for any length of time and excess intakes are excreted, so the diet must include regular supplies. These vitamins also seep out of food into cooking liquids. They are sensitive to heat and light, and the levels in food diminish with staleness.

Even though the fat-soluble vitamins are stored in the body, they are still required regularly but they can be eaten to excess. These vitamins are not as easily lost during food preparation and boiling, but they are lost with fat during roasting, frying and grilling.

Vitamin C is found in fruit and vegetables. It is essential for healthy tissue and known as the vitamin that is vital for good skin. It is necessary for the process of absorbing and utilizing other nutrients, such as iron. Vitamin C is also an antioxidant, helping to protect the body and repair any damage caused by free radicals.

The B-group vitamins are important for the metabolism, the breaking down, absorbing and using of food. They also fulfil other vital tasks, including maintaining a healthy nervous system and generating red blood cells.

Vitamin B1 or **thiamin** is found in meat and offal, wholegrains, nuts, beans and pulses. It is important for the nervous system and in ensuring that the body can release and use energy from food.

Vitamin B2 or **riboflavin** is found in meat, offal, eggs, milk and its products, fish, fortified cereals, and flours. Riboflavin helps the body to release and use energy from food. Riboflavin is light-sensitive – so the content of this vitamin diminishes in milk which is left to stand in the sun.

Niacin or **nicotinic acid** is found in poultry, meat, fish, nuts and vegetables. It is essential for cell function and for passing messages through the nervous system. It is important for the release and use of energy.

Vitamin B6 or **pyridoxine** is found in many foods, including fish, poultry, meat, vegetables, cereals, nuts and yeast extract. It is important for the formation of red blood cells, for a healthy immune system and for breaking down protein.

Vitamin B12 or **cobalamin** is found in animal foods, including fish, poultry, meat, eggs and dairy produce. It is also found in fortified breakfast cereals. This vitamin is essential for producing DNA and so it is vital for all cell generation, including the formation of red blood cells. Since it is widely available in foods, deficiency is rare. However, those following a vegan diet, excluding all animal products, are vulnerable.

Folate or **folic acid** is found in green vegetables, liver, wheatgerm and fortified cereals. It is essential for the production of red blood cells and all DNA. It is particularly important before conception and during pregnancy for the development of the baby.

Pantothenic acid is found in most foods, including meat and offal, vegetables, dried fruit and nuts. It assists in the release of energy and the manufacture of red blood cells, cholesterol and fat.

Fat-Soluble Vitamins

Vitamin A or **retinol** is found in animal foods, such as oily fish, liver, milk and its products, and eggs. Beta carotene is converted into vitamin A in the body: it is found in highly coloured fruit and vegetables, including carrots, red and orange peppers, mango, apricots and green leafy vegetables. Vitamin A is important for healthy eyes and good night vision, as well as cell construction, the mucous membranes in the eyes, and for the respiratory and digestive tracts. Vitamin A promotes healthy skin and is used for general cell building.

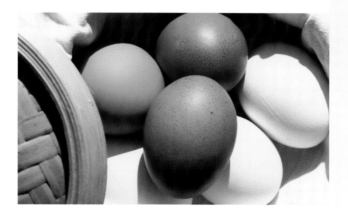

Vitamin D is found in liver, oily fish, eggs and fortified margarines. It is also synthesized in the body during exposure to sunlight. Deficiency is rare, except in those who are confined indoors, such as the elderly. Vitamin D is important for calcium and phosphorus absorption, therefore for healthy bones and teeth.

Vitamin E is found in vegetable fats and oils, including nuts, seeds, oils and avocado. It is an important antioxidant, protecting the body from damage caused by free radicals.

Vitamin K is found in green leafy vegetables. It is important for the normal clotting of the blood.

Minerals

Minerals assist with specific and general functions throughout the body. While some minerals are only required in small amounts, they are still important and the body must have an adequate supply to function well.

Calcium is found in milk and milk products, sardines and other fish where the bones are normally eaten (such as canned salmon), shellfish, dark leafy green vegetables and sesame seeds. Oxalic acid in spinach and phytic acid in the outer layers of whole grains inhibit the absorption of calcium. Vitamin D is also essential for calcium absorption. Calcium is important for healthy bones and teeth.

Copper is found in a wide range of foods and deficiency is rare. Liver, shellfish, nuts and mushrooms all provide copper. It is important for iron absorption, the manufacture of red blood cells and connective tissue, and it helps protect the body against damage from free radicals.

Fluorine is found in fish, although the main dietary source, to varying degrees, is water, depending on soil and local policies on the fluoridation of tap water. It is important for the enamel coating on teeth and for healthy bones but an excess can be damaging, causing the overformation or hardening of bones

Iodine is found in seafood, including seaweed, vegetables and fruit. The level of iodine in food depends on the soil, with more in coastal areas. Iodine is essential in small amounts for a healthy thyroid gland and the levels of hormone it produces to control energy production as well as growth and development. Iodine deficiency leads to an under-active thyroid gland, one of the symptoms of which is a general lack of energy.

Iron is found in meat and offal, egg yolks and green leafy vegetables. Iron from vegetables, such as spinach and watercress, is not as easily absorbed as that from animal sources. Vitamin C aids iron absorption, so it is helpful to combine foods rich in vitamin C with those rich in iron. The body limits the amount of iron that it will absorb and store, so the diet must include a regular supply. Iron is important for haemoglobin or red blood cell production and for the proper functioning of enzymes.

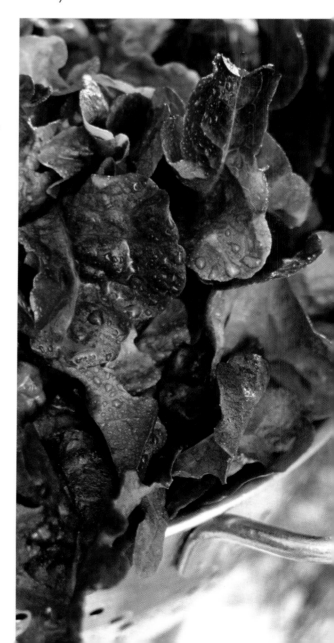

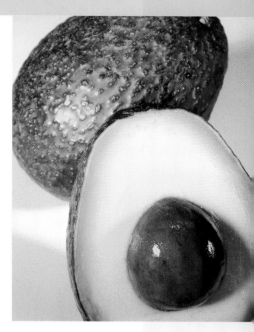

Magnesium is found in dairy produce, grains, pulses, green vegetables and nuts, as well as many other foods. Deficiency is rare in a good, mixed diet. It is important for enzyme activity and the function of the nervous system and muscles.

Manganese is found in plant foods in levels that depend on the amount in the soil. It is obtained from whole grains, pulses and nuts. Its roles include enzyme activity, proper thyroid function, insulin production, and muscle and nerve function. Deficiency is rare in a healthy, mixed diet.

Molybdenum is widely distributed in plant foods and liver, and deficiency is rare. It is important for proper enzyme function.

Phosphorus is found in animal foods, plants and whole grains, and deficiency is rare. It is vital for healthy bones and teeth, and for energy production. It is also found in, and is important to the function of, body proteins. It is so widely available that deficiency is rare but it can be eaten to excess. The phosphorus and calcium in the diet should be balanced, as too much phosphorus can cause the body to reduce its calcium absorption, resulting in calcium deficiency. Phosphorus and calcium are found in the same natural foods; however, phosphorus is found in processed foods in the form of phosphates (compounds of phosphorus), and diets with a high content of processed foods, rich in phosphates but low in calcium, can lead to an imbalance.

Potassium is found in most foods, especially meat, whole grains, vegetables, celery, citrus fruit and bananas. With sodium, potassium is important for bodily fluid balance and efficient nerve and muscle activity.

Selenium is widely available in fish, meat, offal, dairy produce, citrus fruit, grains and avocados. Levels in plant sources relate to those in the soil. Selenium plays roles in hormone activity, growth and development. It is important for healthy eyes and hair, and as an antioxidant, helping to protect against damage from free radicals.

Sodium is found in sodium chloride or salt. It is essential, with potassium, for balancing fluid levels in the body, and for nerve and muscle function. Salt is so widely used that diets can have too high a sodium content, especially when lots of processed and prepared products (generally containing lots of salt) are eaten regularly. A very high salt content contributes to the problem of high blood pressure. Sodium is lost in sweat, so levels have to be replenished.

Sulphur is a compound found in proteins, so it is available from animal foods, fish and pulses. It is important in body proteins, including skin, hair, nails and connective tissue, and vital to many of the body's hormonal functions.

Zinc is found in fish and shellfish, as well as all animal foods and whole grains. Zinc in animal foods is more readily absorbed that that in vegetable sources. It is important for enzyme activity and for the activity of the immune system, as well as for night vision, taste and digestion, and energy production.

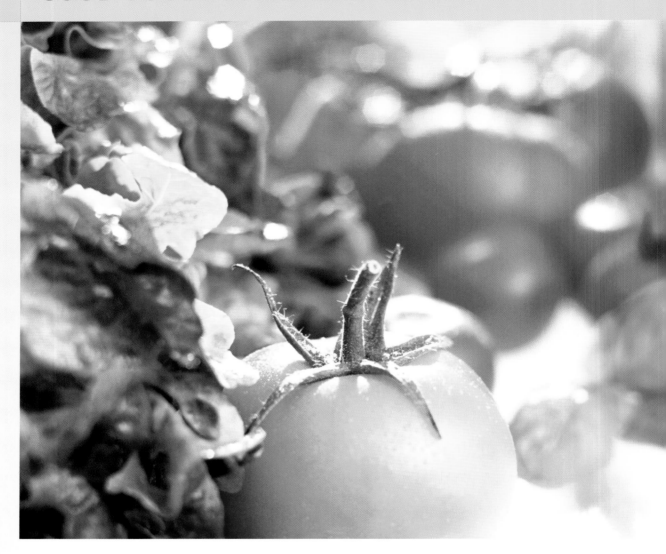

Phytochemicals

In addition to well-documented nutrients, many thousand plant substances contribute to health. Plant chemicals or phytochemicals are thought to protect the body against disease and its causes, particularly against free radicals which latch on to cells in the body or oxidize them.

These phytochemicals include the carotenoids and carotenes. These two are well known, particularly beta carotene, the substance that gives carrots and other vegetables and fruit their strong colour. Lycopene is the carotenoid in tomatoes. Allicin is a substance found in plants of the onion family. A vast group of substances, known as glucosolinates, are found in the crucifera family of vegetables, which includes mustard greens, cabbage, curly kale, Brussels sprouts, broccoli, cauliflower, swede and radishes. Flavonoids or bio-flavonoids include thousands of different substances that are often associated with vegetables with a slightly sweet flavour because they contain glucose compounds. Phytoestrogens are plant chemicals found in a variety of plant foods. They are similar to oestrogen, the female sex hormone, and their activity is similar to that of the hormone.

Promoting a positive state of mind

Including a good mix of foods is essential for bodily health, and emphasizing the different groups that complement mental needs compliments this to maximize diet potential. The following is a guide to matching food to mood.

Calming and soothing

When stress and depression are problems, include foods that are calming and rich in nutrients to support the nervous system. These include the B vitamins, vitamin C, zinc, magnesium, iron and copper. Complex carbohydrates are also important alongside other nutrients.

Fish and seafood are especially positive. Also important are the following fruit and vegetables: apples, apricots, bananas, peaches, pears, asparagus, beetroot, the cabbage family and other green vegetables, celery, potatoes and pumpkins. Include whole cereals, such as oats, and pulses.

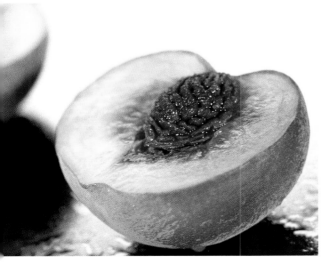

For vitality and vigour

A diet rich in all types of fruit and vegetables is important for antioxidant vitamins, with fruit and vegetable drinks and snacks supplementing the portions included in main meals. Apples, bananas, currants (especially blackcurrants) and strawberries are good examples; try to include lots of mixed fruits in breakfast cereals, desserts and snacks. Carbohydrates are important as an invigorating source of energy – lack of them may be associated with bloating or drowsiness. Dried fruit, such as figs, apricots and prunes, are a good source of natural sugars and fibre.

To restore and boost

When the body is below par it benefits from a mix of styles and dishes, bringing together comforting ingredients and styles, plus foods to boost vitality – so a super supply of fresh fruit and vegetables is essential. The onion family (all types of onions, leeks and garlic) are traditional healers and cure-all ingredients. Nasturtiums – the leaves, seeds and flowers – are a traditional general tonic and good for restoring a run-down mind. Gooseberries, lemons, papayas and rhubarb are all stimulating, while pears are easy on the digestive system.

To comfort and reassure

This shares the same food groups as those for calming and soothing, but with the added requirement for reassurance and familiarity. The recipe section provides a range of recipes that fulfil the need for comfort food, while also making a useful contribution to the diet.

Herbs and spices

As well as main ingredients, herbs and spices are especially useful for their influence on mental wellbeing. Many herbs and spices have ancient medicinal uses and long-established roles in home cures or comforts. The essential oils of many culinary ingredients are used in aromatherapy, with due care and respect for their potency, and it is a good idea to consider the value of aromatherapy and massage in complementing a positive diet for mind and body. In their plant form, herbs and spices are mild and, used regularly in cookery, they can make a positive contribution to the sense of wellbeing.

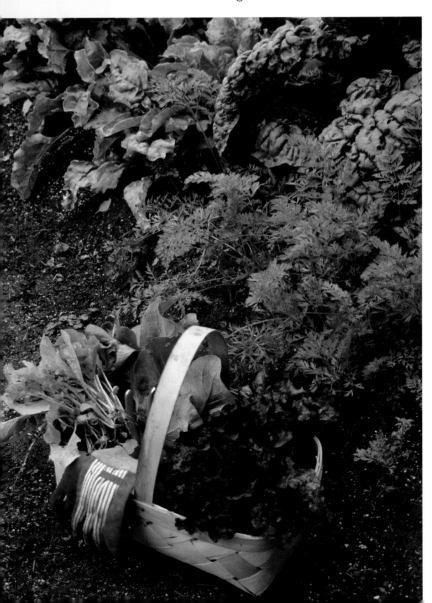

Herbs

Herbs often act as an aid to digestion and they can be balancing in the sense of being either soothing or stimulating.

Angelica Known in cookery as a bright green candied stem most often used to decorate cakes and sweet dishes. Angelica has a fresh 'green' flavour. It grows easily, forming tall, hollow stems with large seed-forming flower heads. The freshly picked stem can be washed and simmered in water to make an infusion for flavouring fruit juices or teas. The seeds and roots are used in herbal medicine and the seeds are used to flavour liqueurs. In herbal medicine, angelica is credited as a great curative. It is said to be a good tonic and stimulant, helpful in the detoxification and cleansing of the body, and for strengthening the immune system.

Basil Its ancient reputation is as a stimulant and uplifting herb but it is also regarded as calming. It is thought to aid digestion and to help ease headaches, migraine, stress and nervous disorders. It has an uplifting flavour.

Bay Widely used to flavour savoury recipes, bay contributes a subtle, spicy warmth to dishes. Bay aids digestion and is traditionally thought to help cure colds and influenza.

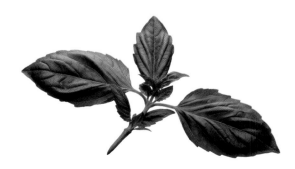

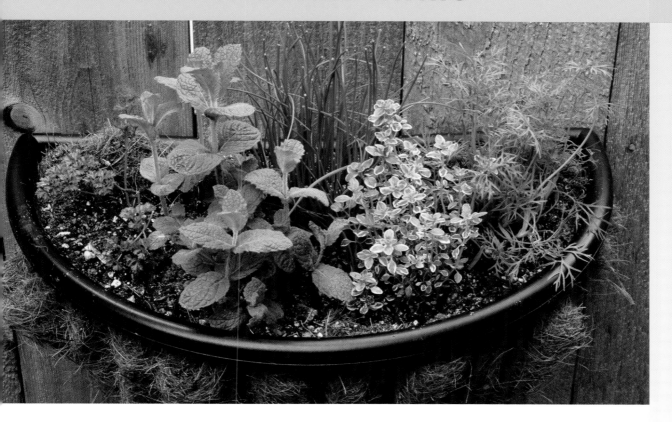

Borage A traditional herb for flavouring summer drinks and salads, borage has an ancient reputation for lifting the spirits. It has diuretic and anti-inflammatory properties, and is said to soothe catarrh and bronchitis.

Camomile Best known for making herb tea, there are several species of camomile. It is known as a calming herb, suitable for aiding sleep, and for easing stomach upsets.

Chervil A cleansing herb, chervil has a reputation for assisting with urinary and liver complaints. It is similar in flavour to, but lighter than, parsley.

Coriander (Cilantro) The leaves are a full-flavoured, quite 'savoury' herb with a powerful, cutting flavour and quite sharp, fresh 'green' aroma. The seeds are of a very different character– mellow and warm in aroma and flavour. Coriander has a reputation for aiding digestion and easing flatulence. It is also thought to stimulate the appetite.

Dill The feathery fronds of the herb have a slightly aniseed flavour. The seeds are used as a spice and they reflect the flavour of the herb but in a subtle and more mature sense. Dill is known for aiding digestion, soothing indigestion and flatulence, and helping sleep. It is an ingredient in gripe water, given to babies suffering from colic.

Elderflower The fabulous aroma and sweet, flowery flavour of elderflower is wonderful in fruit drinks and sweet dishes. Elderflower is traditionally thought of as a cleansing agent, diurectic and gentle laxative. It helps to ease catarrh and is thought to help relieve colds.

Fennel The plant that provides the herb and spice differs from the vegetable in that it does not form the swollen stem base, the fennel bulb used as the vegetable and sometimes referred to as Florence fennel. The herb takes the form of feathery fronds and the seeds are used as a spice. They both have a pronounced aniseed flavour and are popular for herb teas. The vegetable, herb and spice share similar properties, with a reputation for aiding digestion and calming the system. Fennel is said to ease nausea, flatulence and indigestion. It is also a diuretic.

Lavender Lavender is used to flavour some desserts and ices. Its distinctive aroma and flavour complement sweet and fruity dishes. Lavender is appreciated its for many uses: as an antiseptic and anti-bacterial plant, as a way of soothing colds, clearing the head, and easing catarrh. It is a plant with calming and balancing properties, useful for helping relaxation and aiding sleep.

Marjoram and **Oregano** These are warming herbs, with marjoram being the milder and oregano (or wild marjoram as it is sometimes known) being stronger in flavour and properties. Marjoram and oregano are known for their antiseptic properties, useful in aiding the treatment of sore throats. These are calming and sleep-inducing herbs, with warming and comforting properties that ease stress and distress.

Mint There are many varieties of this familiar herb. Mint has a lively aroma and flavour, and it is a popular flavouring in sweet and savoury dishes, and drinks. Mint is thought to aid digestion, calm the stomach, ease flatulence and assist in treating constipation. It has a reputation for being both soothing and stimulating.

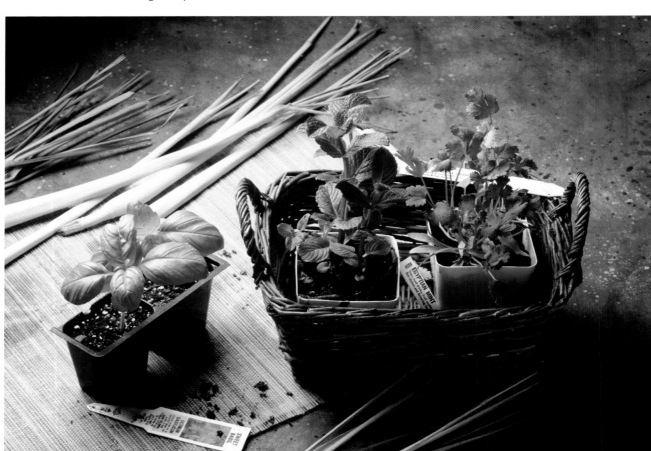

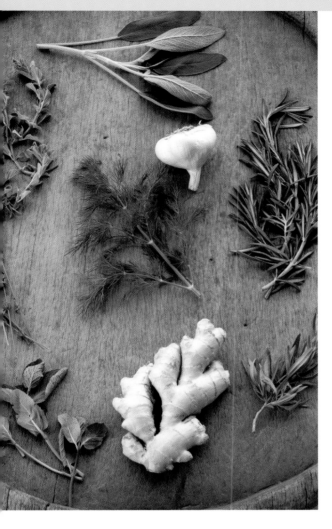

Sage Warm, peppery sage is widely used in savoury cooking. Its very familiarity is comforting. Traditionally, sage is thought of as a tonic and a healing herb. It is thought to be useful for calming nerves as well as stimulating the nervous system. It is said to promote good circulation. It was also used traditionally to stimulate menstruation.

Tarragon Tarragon is a tender, fresh-tasting herb with a strong aniseed flavour (French tarragon is the herb cultivated for culinary use; Russian tarragon has little flavour). Tarragon is a used as an aid to digestion and for easing flatulence and nausea. It is has also been used to soothe toothache.

Thyme Strongly aromatic and with a warm flavour, thyme is widely used in savoury cooking. It has a reputation as an antiseptic helpful in the treatment of sore throats and mouth infections. Thyme is also said to stimulate the appetite and aid digestion. Thyme is another of the herbs that is thought to have a balancing effect – on the one hand it is stimulating but it can also help to calm stress and therefore assist with sleep and relaxation.

Parsley Parsley is a cleansing herb, with a reputation for neutralizing strong smells. It is a mild diuretic and is thought to help regulate the menstrual cycle. It also aids digestion and relieves flatulence.

Rosemary Full-flavoured rosemary is widely used in savoury cookery and excellent for making herb tea. It has a reputation as an antiseptic. The flavour and aroma is warm and rosemary oil is stimulating, thought to benefit the nervous system and brain. Rosemary is a head-clearing herb, for easing headaches as well as helping with the congestion associated with colds. It is also thought to be a general tonic and may even help in the lowering of the body's cholesterol levels.

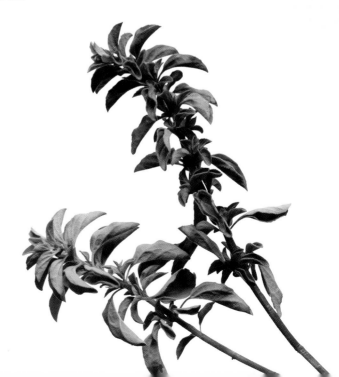

Spices

Spices are usually more potent than their related herbs, both in flavour and in benefits, because they are usually derived from the seeds or other parts of the plant that contain a higher concentration of essential plant substances. As with herbs, spices are traditional aids to digestion and are known particularly for relieving or helping to prevent flatulence, for example, when combined with pulses.

Aniseed Aniseed has a strong flavour, appreciated in baking, in European cookery, and as one of the ingredients in Chinese five-spice powder. It is also used to flavour drinks and liqueurs, such as Greek ouzo and French Pernod. It has a reputation for stimulating the appetite, aiding digestion and relieving flatulence. It was also used as a traditional comfort for coughs, colds and asthma, and in soothing potions for helping sleep.

Caraway Caraway seeds have a warm flavour that goes well with all sorts of fruit, especially in warm drinks. Caraway is warming and comforting, related to dill and fennel. It stimulates the appetite, aids digestion and relieves flatulence.

Cardamoms Aromatic, refreshing and head-clearing, cardamoms are reminiscent of citrus and eucalyptus. They are said to aid digestion and settle the stomach as well as refresh the breath. Cardamoms help to clear the head and make soothing drinks for those suffering from colds and influenza.

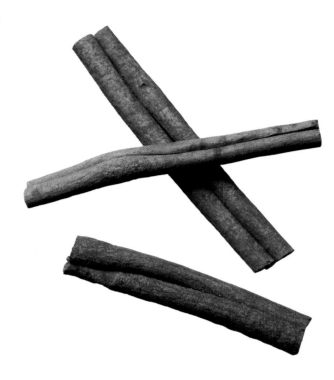

Cinnamon Warming cinnamon helps to clear the head, so it is a helpful spice to include in cold-cure drinks. It is also believed to help aid digestion, relieve flatulence and promote circulation.

Cloves Cloves have an affinity for apples and are a classic spice for making warming mulled drinks – just as good with apple, pear or grape juice as with wine. Best known as a home-cure for toothache, cloves possess anaesthetic and antiseptic qualities. Cloves are a stimulant, an aid to digestion and can relieve flatulence.

Coriander (Cilantro) As for the herb, coriander is thought of as a stimulant and an aid to digestion.

Cumin Said to stimulate the appetite. It is diuretic and a stimulant.

Dill Dill seeds are the spice from the dill plant. See herbs.

Fennel Fennel seeds are the spice from the fennel plant. See herbs.

Ginger Ginger is available as the fresh root; preserved in syrup or candied; as the dried root; or dried and ground to a powder. Fresh root ginger tastes terrific with all sorts of dishes. Ginger is known for easing nausea and helping to ease diarrhoea. It is said to promote sweating and good circulation, as well helping to fight against infection when used as a cold-cure drink.

Juniper Little dark berries – almost black – used for bringing a rich flavour to game, poultry and meat in cooking. It is one of the flavouring ingredients in gin. Known as a diuretic and antiseptic, juniper is a cleansing spice, used to promote detoxication and as a tonic. It is also an appetite stimulant.

Mustard Mustard is warming, known for traditional use in poultices and hot mustard baths. It goes well with tomato juice and mixtures of vegetable juices , and is used to make warming, comforting drinks and soups to soothe the symptoms of colds.

Nutmeg and **Mace** Warm spices that aid digestion, act as a stimulant and a tonic. They can ease nausea and flatulence. In large quantities, these spices can cause drowsiness and hallucinations and even be poisonous, but in the small amounts used in cookery, this is not the case.

Turmeric Bright yellow in colour, with an earthy, yet refreshing, flavour, turmeric has a reputation as a tonic, a stimulant, an anti-bacterial and anti-septic spice.

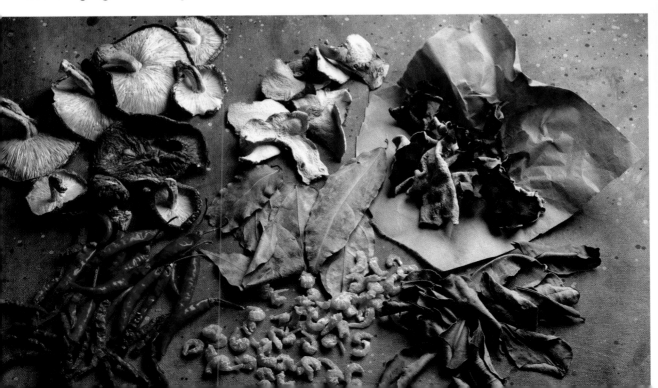

The following collection of recipes is intended to inspire and encourage a positive approach to food, cooking and eating. They are grouped in chapters according to their potential for helping to counteract everyday problems and balance a healthy mind and body.

Check-up time

In physical terms, the approach is extremely healthy, providing all the nutrients the body needs to be super-fit. However, if you have any doubts about your health – physical or mental – consult your doctor for advice. Diet and a positive outlook are excellent for putting life into perspective and lifting the spirits, and eating the right foods certainly helps to avoid or overcome minor everyday ailments. However, illness should never be overlooked in the hope that gentle changes to eating habits will sort a problem. In any case, it is a good idea to have a general health check occasionally, especially if the world is seeming too much, or before embarking on a change of lifestyle, diet or activity.

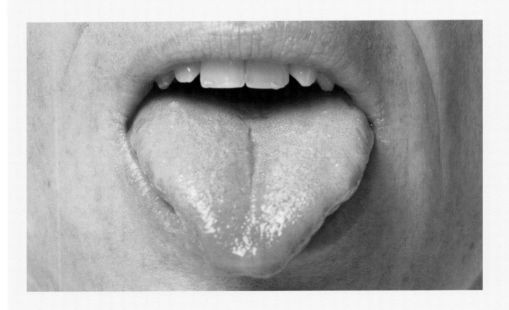

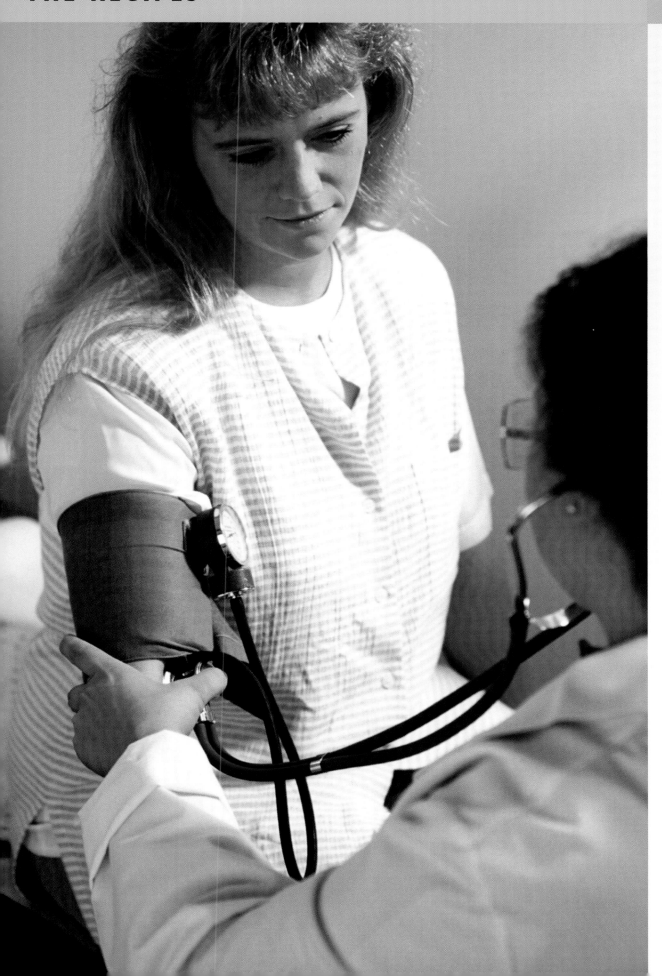

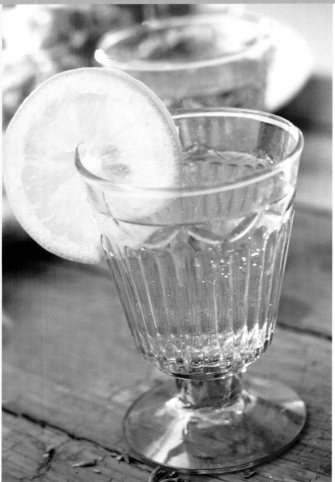

Moving on from detoxification to adopting a different approach to shopping, food, cooking and eating may be an overnight one-stop decision for someone living alone with a strong will and oodles of enthusiasm but it is more practical to introduce a new regime step-by-step. This may be by making a move on one meal a day, or aiming for a regular shopping trip to re-think food ideas. Making a realistic plan is a good idea, especially when other members of the household are affected – and remember to involve them and enlist their support.

Children should not be subjected to diet restrictions that are likely to impair their nourishment. The best way to encourage youngsters is to inspire them with a positive, fun approach to cooking and eating – never negative.

Make a change

For best results, changes in diet and lifestyle should be gradual, especially when it involves others or if you are trying to instill a new approach within the family. On a personal level – or for other adults – a phase of detoxification is an excellent starting point for clearing and cleansing the system. However, remember that some aspects of this must be gradual. For example, cutting out caffeine-rich drinks is fine if they are only consumed on a one- or two-a-day basis, but if several are drunk then stopping them all at once is likely to produce withdrawal symptoms. So cut down before cutting out. Similarly, excess alcohol should be reduced and removed, and smoking is a definite no-no to be overcome. Drinking plenty of water is important.

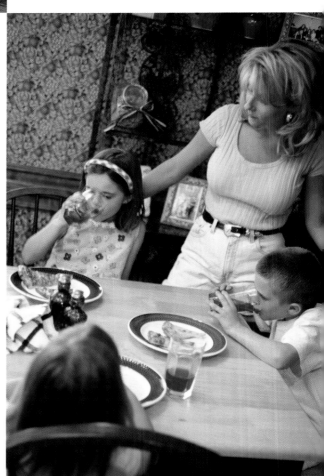

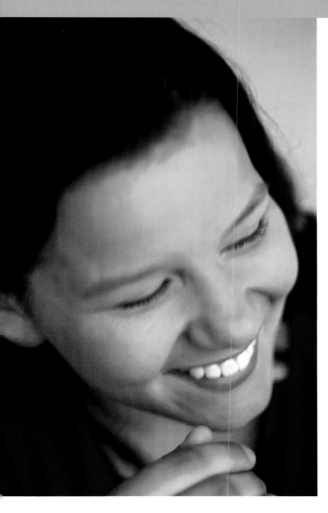

Relaxation is the other vital ingredient for a healthy outlook on life. This means different things to different people. Many lively and energetic individuals cringe at the mention of the word, which conjures up for them ideas of serious yoga or mind-emptying meditation, but it does not have to be like that at all. Mind emptying is important – there is nothing worse for stress than an over-filled brain positively prickling as ideas shoot across and concerns are sparked at an alarming rate per second. How you choose to switch off is for you to decide – it may be by classic relaxation techniques (on which there are many books and tapes), by walking (an excellent way to loosen limbs gently and take in surroundings while letting stress dissipate slightly) or by engaging in some kind of activity or sport. While some find complete and absorbing mental distraction the way to empty their heads of the everyday issues that generate stress, others prefer to relax physically and concentrate on the head-emptying process. Talking to others may be another means of alleviating stress and relaxing.

Humour the healer

One of the best ways to relax, revitalize and get a new perspective is to exercise the sense of humour. However difficult it may seem, find the catalyst that triggers your sense of humour because there is nothing quite like laughing to relieve stress, promote a sense of wellbeing and bring back the love of life. Laugh and others will share your pleasure – and generate a wonderful sense of wellbeing.

Complementing good diet

A good and vital outlook on mind and body results from more than food alone. Exercise is important – find something that suits you, starting with gentle activity if you are not physically fit (in consultation with your doctor) and gearing this towards the family if you want to involve those around you. Fresh air is a great antidote to all sorts of difficult issues and definitely worth rediscovering if you have forgotten about walking or doing something outside. Something as simple as a good change in routine can make all the difference – eating out occasionally, reading, listening to the radio or talking instead of watching television, or going to the theatre, cinema or an exhibition can be uplifting.

TO CLEAR AND CLEANSE

There seems to be universal acknowledgement of the fact that we all live life at one hundred and ten per cent, but getting down to addressing the problems resulting from this frantic pace requires more than a moment's thought. Firstly, we may have to realise that the 'pace' is not always a physical one but a process of mental rallying that goes unnoticed more easily until it results in physical as well as mental fatigue, if not exhaustion.

Beginning with a gentle and practical attitude to clearing and cleansing the physical system couples well with thinking about our state of mind. Thinking about what the food we eat – or the quantity in which we eat it – does to the body, is part of the process of caring. This is often associated with the individual urge to lose weight but that does not have to be the case: taking a positive look at one's own eating habits, a joint diet with a partner or for a whole family, is an excellent way of promoting a positive attitude.

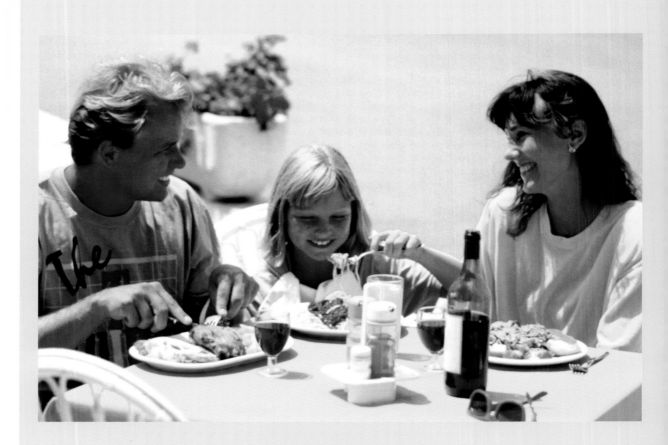

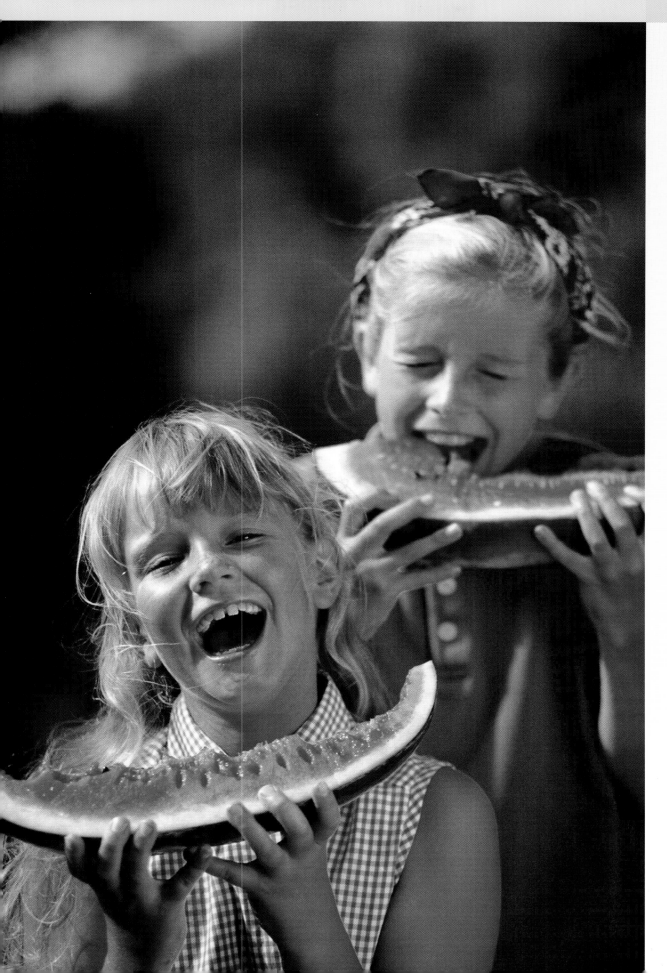

So what does this cleansing mean and why is it worthwhile? This is not about losing weight – even if the long-term aim is to lose weight to a healthy level. The first stage is to feel better physically and mentally. Everyday diet is often neglected in a busy lifestyle: several snacks replace one proper meal; processed products take over from simple foods; the balance of nutrients may be poor; and meal times may barely exist as eating becomes another hassle. Drinking too much tea, coffee or alcohol and too little water does not help. The body works to capacity to digest and clear out the waste products from a poor diet – the kidneys and liver have to cope with all the toxins that the body takes in, excreting them to avoid a build-up.

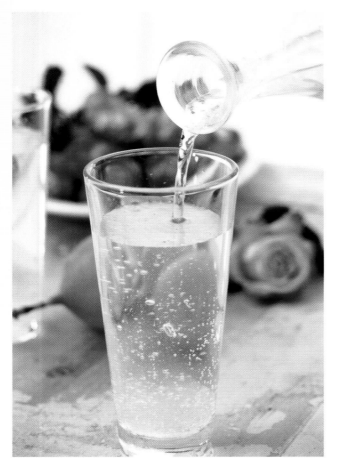

Fasting is sometimes advocated as a good way of beginning the process of detoxification. There are many opinions on, and ways of practising, fasting, ranging from replacing individual meals with fresh fruit, vegetables or water, to building up to regularly cutting out food on a daily basis. While taking a day off to relax and reduce food intake to a minimum – or even to concentrate on fruit and vegetable drinks supplemented by plenty of water – can be a good idea, indulging in any prolonged or frequent fasting is not to be recommended. The negative side of fasting cannot be overstressed – it cuts out essential nutrients required by the body; it can lead to a process of starving and overeating; and it will not produce a genuine, mid- to long-term sense of wellbeing. There is a danger that fasting can become a way of exercising self-control that can lead to a negative view of food, and to the eating disorders associated with that. Fasting should never be imposed on others, especially in terms of family eating.

Instead of taking a negative 'no food' kind of approach, the better method is to think about introducing good things to the diet. Cleansing or detoxifying means cutting out the products and drinks that tend to overload the system, and concentrating on eating positive foods and ingredients that help to clear the build-up of toxins in the body. Adopting this positive focus is extremely good for the mind as well as the body, and combining this approach to eating with a general appraisal of fitness, relaxation and exercise ,is ideal. That does not necessarily mean a major lifestyle review or indulging in a frantic new regime. Simply allowing a few minutes every day to think about some form of suitable relaxation is a great starting point. On the food front, the guidelines are simple.

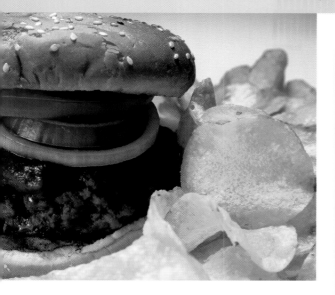

Move on to the positive points.

- Focus on eating plenty of fruit and vegetables – fresh and frozen are both fine.

- Include lots of raw fruit and vegetables as snacks, salads or in composite dishes.

- Include fish, poultry and vegetarian meals as the main focus, so as to have some meat-free days.

- Drink plenty of water.

- Drink plenty of fruit or vegetable juice.

- Include enough complex carbohydrate and fibre to provide a ready source of energy and avoid constipation, but try to avoid a stodgy diet.

- Concentrate on ingredients, herbs and spices that are thought to aid digestion and cleanse the system.

Dispense with the negative aspects quickly and simply.

- Cut down on processed foods and convenience foods.

- Avoid alcohol.

- Cut out or reduce tea and coffee intake.

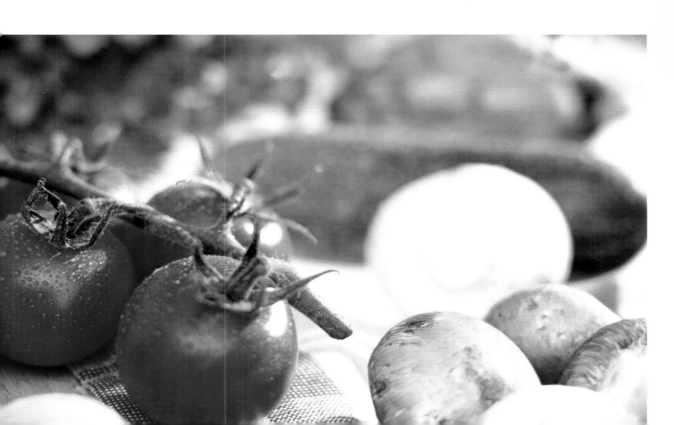

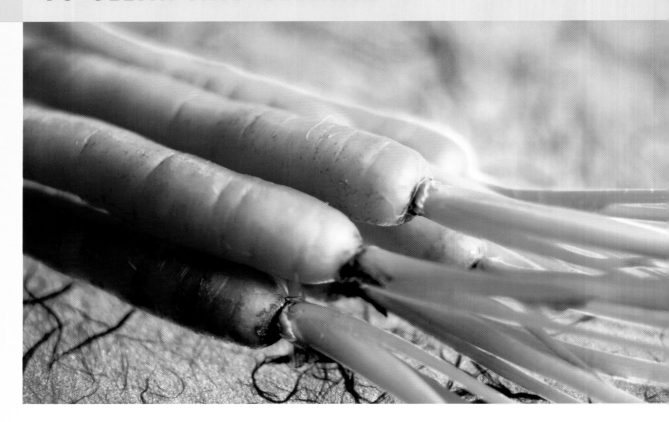

Orange-scented Carrot and Celery Soup

Zingy orange and sweet carrots are a classic and successful combination as their flavours balance each other perfectly. In this recipe celery contributes a slightly peppery twist to the soup. Packed with beta carotene, vitamin C and minerals, the soup is helpful in cleansing and clearing the system. Celery is thought to help lower blood pressure, assist in reducing water retention and promote kidney function, thus helping to cleanse the system.

Serves 6

2 tablespoons olive oil
1 large onion, chopped
4 celery sticks (stalks), sliced
salt and pepper
450 g/1 lb carrots, sliced
1 medium potato, coarsely diced
900 ml/1½ pints/3¾ cups vegetable or chicken stock
2 large, juicy oranges

Place the olive oil in a large saucepan and add the onion and celery. Add a little salt and pepper, keeping the salt to a minimum. Cover and cook over medium heat for about 20 minutes, or until the vegetables are softened but not browned.

Add the carrots, potato and stock. Grate the rind from 1 orange and add it to the pan with the stock. Bring to the boil, reduce the heat and cover the pan. Simmer the soup for 30 minutes, until the vegetables are tender.

Purée the soup in a blender until smooth, then return it to the saucepan and add the orange juice. Reheat, stirring occasionally, and serve. Alternatively, the soup tastes good chilled – allow it to cool completely, chilling it for several hours before serving.

Spinach and Basil Broth with Prawns

This aromatic broth is deliciously light and ideal for promoting a sense of healthy eating and wellbeing. Along with other shellfish, prawns provide a good source of protein, vitamin B12, iodine and selenium. Selenium may help in a detox diet by binding with unwanted toxins (metals) and flushing them out of the system. Spinach is a valuable source of folate and basil is an uplifting herb which has long been thought of as a natural tonic and aid to digestion.

Serves 4

2 garlic cloves, chopped
1 thin slice of peeled fresh ginger root, finely chopped
1 bunch of spring onions (scallions), thinly sliced
2 pieces lemon grass
900 ml/1½ pints/3¾ cups chicken stock
salt and pepper
450 g/1 lb raw peeled tiger prawns
225 g/8 oz spinach, finely shredded
25 g/1 oz tender basil sprigs and leaves
handful of fresh coriander (cilantro)

Place the garlic, ginger, spring onions and lemon grass in a saucepan. Pour in the stock and heat gently until simmering. Cover the pan and simmer for 15 minutes. Taste the stock and add a little salt, if necessary, and pepper.

Add the prawns to the simmering stock and poach them gently for about 5 minutes, or until they are pink and cooked. Do not allow the stock to boil rapidly or overcook the prawns as they will become tough. Use a draining spoon to remove the prawns from the pan.

Add the spinach to the soup and bring back to the boil. Cover and simmer for 5 minutes. Meanwhile, chop half the prawns. Replace the chopped and whole prawns and heat for a few seconds without boiling. Shred the basil and coriander and add to the soup – the easiest way to do this is with scissors, straight into the pan. Remove from the heat and serve immediately.

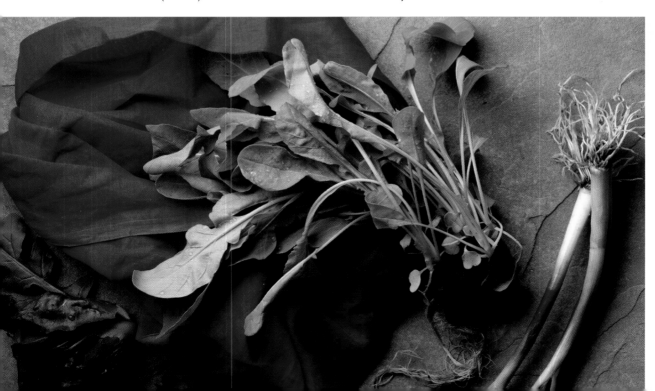

Grilled Plaice with Asparagus and Avocado in Parsley Dressing

White fish is light and appealing in a cleansing diet. Both asparagus and parsley are traditionally regarded as tonics, helping to aid digestion and acting as diuretics. This dish provides a good cross-section of nutrients ranging from the protein, minerals and vitamins from the fish and asparagus, to the vitamin E and potassium from the creamy avocado. Serve new potatoes to complete the light meal.

Serves 4

225 g/8 oz asparagus spears (stalks)
4 large white-skinned plaice fillets
5 tablespoons olive oil
salt and pepper
grated rind and juice of ½ lemon
large bunch of parsley, finely chopped
bunch of chives, finely snipped
2 avocados

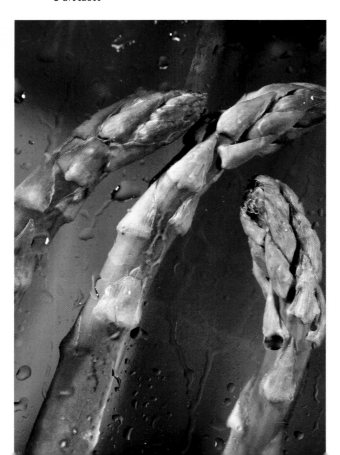

Trim any tough or woody stalk ends off the asparagus, leaving just the tender spears. (The stalk ends can be used in stock for soup.) Cook the spears in a roasting tin or large frying pan of simmering, salted water for 5 minutes, or until just tender. The time depends on the size and age of spears: while tender young spears will cook in about 5 minutes, older, larger spears can take up to 10 minutes. Drain the asparagus.

Preheat the grill on the hottest setting. Remove any stray bones from the fish fillets and place them skin side up on a foil-lined grill rack. Brush the skin with a little oil and grill close to the heat source until browned. Use a fish slice to turn the fillets. Season the fillets lightly, then lay the asparagus on top, leaving some of the fish uncovered (place excess spears to one side of the pan). Brush with a little oil and grill until the asparagus is browned in places and the fish is just cooked.

Meanwhile, heat the remaining olive oil with the lemon rind and juice in a large saucepan until hot. Whisk in a little seasoning, then remove from the heat and whisk in the parsley and chives. Halve, stone, peel and slice the avocados, adding the slices to the pan of dressing as they are ready.

Transfer the plaice and asparagus to warmed plates and add the avocado slices, spooning over the parsley dressing. Serve at once.

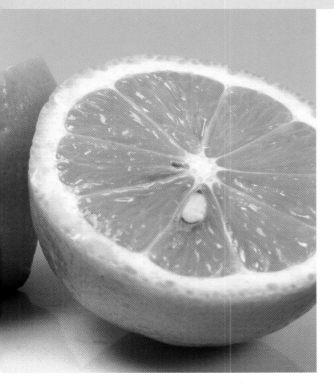

<u>Serves 2</u>

125 g/4 oz can mackerel fillets in olive oil
grated rind and juice of ½ lemon
100 g/4 oz/1 cup rye flakes
1 garlic clove, chopped
2 spring onions (scallions), chopped
2 celery sticks (stalks), diced
⅓ cucumber, diced
freshly ground black pepper
large handful of tender parsley sprigs, very coarsely chopped

Drain all the oil from the can of mackerel into a bowl. Whisk in the lemon rind and juice. Add the rye flakes and garlic and mix thoroughly to coat all the flakes in the oil and lemon dressing.

Quick Mackerel and Rye Salad

Making the connection with positive, feel-good eating is easy once you are tuned in to the approach – and that means having a few practical food ideas to make the most of good ingredients. This is a simple storecupboard salad: it is assembled in minutes, tastes terrific and makes you feel good. Rather than shun canned ingredients completely when cleansing the system, it is more sensible to be selective and make life easier to promote a positive attitude to food. Canned mackerel in olive oil is a good source of omega-3 fatty acids. Since salt is added, the salad does not need extra seasoning and the oil from the can makes a good dressing. Diced celery, garlic, spring onions and parsley all help the cleansing process.

Mix in the spring onions, celery and cucumber and season with freshly ground black pepper to taste. Flake the mackerel and add it to the salad with the parsley. Fork the fish and parsley into the grain mixture and serve.

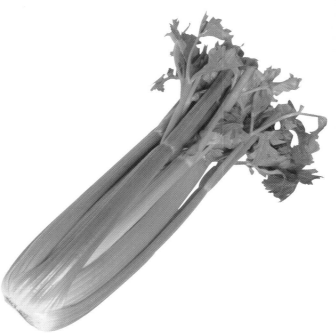

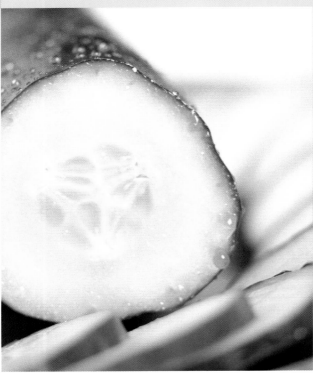
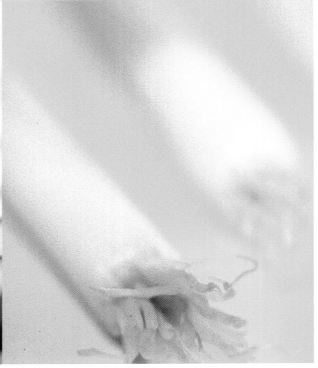

Aromatic Chicken Parcels

Lean chicken is a good choice for light main dishes. Instead of opting for a rich cooking method, the chicken is steamed with cucumber, broccoli and aromatic tarragon and mint. The result is a dish rich in vitamins and cleansing vegetables, with tarragon and mint to stimulate and aid the digestive system.

Serves 4

225 g/8 oz small broccoli florets
1 cucumber
1 spring onion (scallion), chopped
4 small skinless, boneless chicken breasts
4 tablespoons chopped mint, plus 4 large mint sprigs
2 tablespoons chopped tarragon, plus 4 tarragon sprigs
juice of ½ lemon
2 tablespoons olive oil
salt and pepper

Add the broccoli to boiling water, bring back to a full boil, then drain. Peel the cucumber and cut it into 2.5 cm/1 in lengths, then cut these into quarters lengthwise. Mix the broccoli, cucumber and spring onion.

Prepare a saucepan or wok of boiling water and steamer to fit over it. Cut 4 double-thick pieces of foil, each large enough to hold a piece of chicken and a quarter of the vegetables. Place a sprig of mint and tarragon on each piece of foil and lay a chicken breast on top. Arrange the vegetables on the chicken, then season lightly. Sprinkle with the lemon juice and olive oil and fold up the foil tightly to enclose the ingredients in neat, sealed parcels.

Place the chicken parcels in the steamer. Cook over steadily boiling water for 40 minutes. Open the top of one parcel carefully and use the point of a knife to check that the chicken is cooked before removing all the parcels from the steamer. Open the tops of the parcels and sprinkle with the chopped mint and tarragon. Serve at once.

Soya Bean and Fennel Salad with Coriander and Orange

Soya beans are an excellent source of protein and a great alternative to fish, poultry or meat. They are small, firm and delicate in flavour, and absolutely delicious with crisp aniseed-scented fennel, pungent coriander and refreshing orange in this salad. Coriander and fennel are both positive ingredients to include in a detoxification programme, as are oranges for their useful vitamin C content. Cutting out red meat and opting for mainly vegetarian meals helps to kick-start the body into a new and positive approach to food and diet.

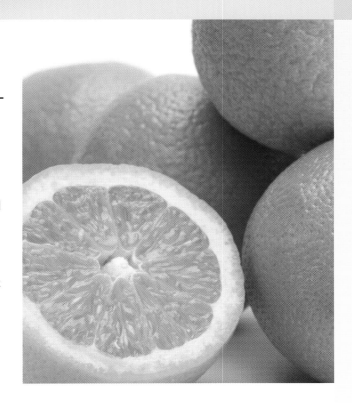

Serves 2

2 oranges
salt and pepper
2 tablespoons walnut oil
100 g/14 oz can soya beans, rinsed and drained
1 fennel bulb, diced
4 tablespoons snipped chives
150 g/5 oz tender watercress sprigs
handful of coriander (cilantro) leaves

Grate the rind and juice from 1 orange and place them in a bowl. Cut a thin slice off both ends of the remaining orange, then cut off all the peel and pith down the sides. Holding the orange over the bowl to catch any juice, use a small sharp knife to cut the segments from between the membranes, setting them aside on a plate as they are removed.

Whisk a little seasoning into the orange rind and juice, then whisk in the walnut oil. Add the soya beans, fennel and chives, and stir well. Mix the watercress and coriander, then divide the leaves between four bowls. Add the orange segments to the soya beans and fennel and mix lightly. Spoon the mixture on to the watercress and coriander salads. Serve at once.

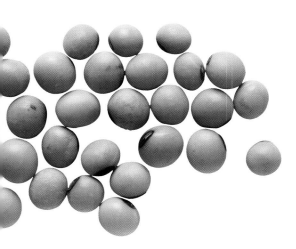

Buckwheat and Red Pepper Salad

Roasted buckwheat, also known as kasha, is popular in Polish and Russian cooking, and dark buckwheat flour is used to make yeasted pancakes or blini. Buckwheat also features as an ingredient in Japanese soba noodles. Buckwheat is one of the foods that may help to reduce high blood pressure; combined with lightly roasted red peppers and juicy tomatoes, it makes a salad rich in antioxidants to help clear the system of a build-up of unwanted toxins. Most importantly, this salad is highly aromatic with marjoram and mint, delicious and satisfying.

Serves 4

175 g/6 oz/1 cup roasted buckwheat
2 tablespoons olive oil
2 large red (bell) peppers, quartered lengthwise and seeded
1 onion, halved and thinly sliced
2 garlic cloves, thinly sliced
1 teaspoon dried marjoram
6 ripe tomatoes, diced
½ teaspoon sugar
salt and pepper
4 tablespoons chopped mint
1 Cos lettuce, separated into leaves, to serve

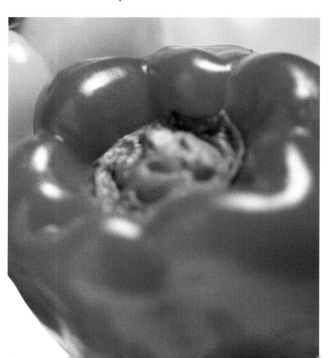

Place the buckwheat in a sieve and rinse it under plenty of cold water. Drain and transfer to a saucepan. Add 450 ml/¾ pint/2 cups water and bring to the boil. Remove the pan from the heat as soon as the water boils. Cover the pan and set it aside for 30 minutes, until all the water has been absorbed and the buckwheat is tender.

Meanwhile, heat the olive oil in a heavy frying pan (skillet) or griddle. Add the peppers, skin sides down, and press them on to the pan. Cook for a few minutes until the pieces are lightly browned, then turn and cook the second sides. The peppers should be slightly tender, but not softened, and browned in places. Remove from the pan and cut across into short strips. Place the pepper strips in a bowl.

Add the onion, garlic and marjoram to the pan. Toss briefly to separate the onion slices into shreds and brown them slightly. Do not cook the onion for too long as the shreds should remain crisp. Add the onion and garlic to the peppers, scraping all the juices and marjoram from the pan. Leave to cool slightly.

Stir the tomatoes, sugar and seasoning into the pepper mixture, then add the mint. Check that the buckwheat has absorbed all the water – if not, drain it in a sieve – then add it to the vegetables and use two forks to lightly mix all the ingredients. Take care not to crush the buckwheat and make it starchy. Serve with Cos lettuce so that the leaves can be used to scoop up the buckwheat salad.

Beetroot, Orange and Papaya Salad

Try this refreshing salad for a light lunch, with slices of sesame and sunflower seed bread, or have it with grilled fish for a fabulous main course. If you start by boiling raw beetroot, then you may want to serve the salad warm as the freshly cooked beet is quite superlative with the zesty orange and smooth papaya, but bought vacuum-packed natural beetroot is perfectly good. The beetroot provides plenty of folate and potassium, as well as vitamin C. The mineral content of beetroot (magnesium, phosphorus and manganese as well as potassium) contribute to the traditional reputation it has as a vegetable to cleanse the blood and stimulate the system. Papaya aids digestion and detoxification, and orange contributes vitamin C as well as a light dressing for this zesty salad.

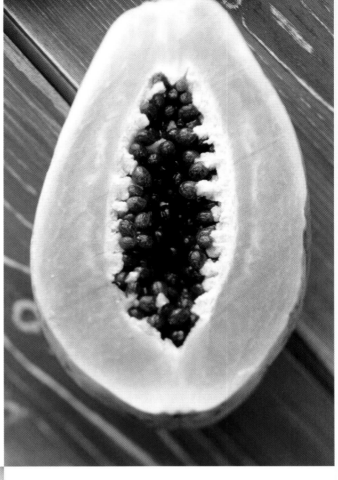

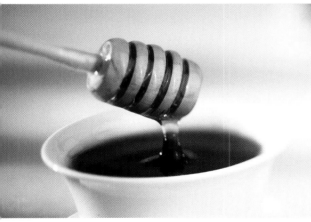

Serves 2

225 g/8 oz cooked beetroot, diced
1 papaya, halved, seeded, peeled and diced
2 oranges
freshly ground black pepper
good pinch of ground ginger
1 teaspoon clear honey
1 teaspoon cider vinegar

Divide the beetroot among two plates or wide, shallow bowls. Add the papaya, sprinkling the dice evenly over the beetroot.

Grate the rind from ½ orange and place it in a bowl, then squeeze the juice from the orange and add it to the rind. Cut all the peel and pith off the second orange, then slice it thinly, discarding any pips. Cut the slices across in half and then into quarters. Sprinkle these over the salads and season with freshly ground black pepper.

Add the ginger to the orange juice, then stir in the honey and cider vinegar. Spoon this dressing over the salads and serve.

New Potato Salad with Cucumber and Shredded Seaweed

Cucumber has a high water content and its gentle, diuretic properties are welcome for detoxifying the system. New potatoes are satisfying, light in flavour and they (along with other potatoes) also help in the process of cleansing. Seaweed is a particularly interesting ingredient, valued as a source of minerals and iodine in particular, needed for the thyroid function. Seaweed is thought to be a cleansing ingredient. The high sodium content of seaweed complements the delicate cucumber and potatoes to make a delicious, satisfying salad. Pepped with just a hint of lemon and fresh root ginger, this salad has an immediate feel-good effect.

Serves 4

15 g/½ oz/½ cup dried shredded hijiki seaweed
1 tablespoon light soy sauce
1 slice fresh root ginger, peeled and finely chopped
1 garlic clove, thinly sliced
grated rind and juice of 1 lemon
250 ml/8 fl oz/1 cup unsweetened apple juice
½ teaspoon sesame oil
675 g/1½ lb small new or salad potatoes
1 cucumber
handful of coriander (cilantro) leaves, coarsely chopped

Place the seaweed in a bowl and pour in boiling water to cover, then leave to soak for 15 minutes. Drain and place in a saucepan. Add the soy sauce, ginger, garlic, lemon rind and juice, apple juice and sesame oil.

Bring to the boil, then reduce the heat and simmer, uncovered, for about 30 minutes, or until the hijiki is tender and glossy and the liquid has virtually evaporated. Stir occasionally and keep an eye on the seaweed towards the end of cooking to ensure it does not dry up completely. Remove from the heat and leave to cool until warm – there should be enough liquid to form a moist dressing for the salad.

Cook the potatoes in boiling water for about 10 minutes, or until tender. Drain the potatoes and cut them in half or into quarters, then divide them among four bowls. Peel and dice the cucumber and sprinkle it over the potatoes. Top with the hijiki, scraping all the juice from the pan and trickling it over, then sprinkle with the coriander.

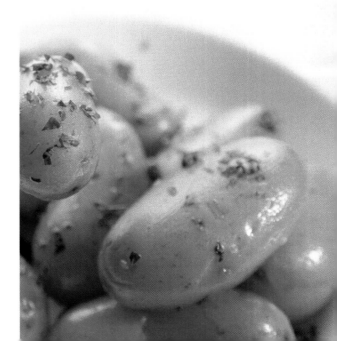

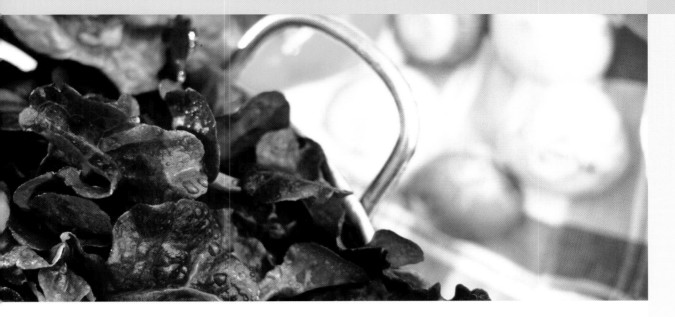

Parsley, Rocket and Nasturtium Leaf Salad with Roasted Fennel Seed Dressing

Serves 2

Serve this light, spirit-lifting salad as a base or accompaniment with grilled fish or seafood, new potatoes or lightly roasted vegetables. It is a real tonic for the system, especially the parsley and nasturtium, both renowned for their cleansing properties, and peppery rocket with its valuable vitamin C content. Roasted fennel seeds bring a fabulous aniseed flavour to the dressing and contribute their own detox characteristics to the salad – this is an especially good salad for cleansing the system of the negative influence of alcohol. The quantities here are not terribly precise because it is the sort of salad to eat in generous proportions – just add handfuls or bagfuls of the leafy ingredients in equal proportions. Tender young dandelion leaves are also good in the salad.

1 tablespoon fennel seeds
2 tablespoons cider vinegar
salt and pepper
1 teaspoon wholegrain mustard
1 teaspoon honey
2 tablespoons olive oil
about 2 large handfuls each of parsley leaves, rocket leaves and nasturtium leaves

Roast the fennel seeds in a small, heavy saucepan over a medium heat until they are aromatic. Immediately tip them into a salad bowl to prevent them from overcooking and becoming bitter.

Add the cider vinegar, a little salt and pepper, the mustard and honey to the fennel seeds. Whisk until thoroughly combined, then whisk in the olive oil to make a slightly thickened dressing.

Add the parsley and rocket leaves to the bowl with any small nasturtium leaves. Use scissors to coarsely shred larger nasturtium leaves. Lightly toss the salad and serve immediately.

Minted Kiwi and Ginger Smoothie

A smoothie makes a great start to the day, an excellent end-of-afternoon snack or a soothing and refreshing drink to go with lunch. The combination of ingredients in this simple smoothie will help to clear the system of toxins and bring a welcome vitamin C boost. Ginger stimulates the system to encourage cleansing. It also helps to ease digestive disorders and wind, useful during a change in diet, especially when increasing the intake of complex carbohydrate and fibre.

Serves 1

2 kiwi fruit, peeled and quartered
1 tablespoon chopped fresh root ginger
1 teaspoon clear honey
1 sprig of mint
250 ml/8 fl oz/1 cup plain yogurt, chilled

Place the kiwi fruit, ginger, honey and leaves from the mint in a blender and process until puréed. Add the yogurt and whizz briefly, then pour the smoothie into a glass and drink.

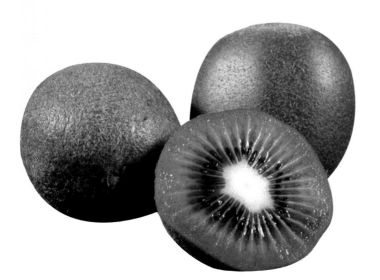

Elderflower and Strawberry Oat Drink

This has a texture of a dairy drink but the creamy result is created using oats instead of milk or yogurt. Strawberries are a classic purifying fruit and elderflower is also a gentle diuretic that aids detoxification. Oats are a good source of carbohydrate and believed to promote a healthy circulatory system. Frozen strawberries can be used instead of fresh, and dried elderflowers are available from some healthfood shops. It is worth making a concentrated infusion of elderflowers in water and freezing it in ice cube trays for winter use. This drink is ideal for breakfast – especially if you leave the elderflowers to infuse in a covered container in the fridge overnight.

Serves 1

1 head of elderflowers
150 ml/¼ pint/⅔ cup boiling water
3 tablespoons rolled oats
150 g/5 oz/⅔ cup strawberries, hulled
1 teaspoon clear honey, or to taste

Pick over the elderflower head carefully to make sure it is clean and free from insects, then rinse it in cold water and shake off the excess. Snip the flowers into a bowl and pour in the boiling water. Cover and leave to infuse for 1 hour, stirring occasionally, or overnight.

Strain the elderflower water and discard the flower heads. In a blender, purée the scented water with the oats, strawberries and honey until it has become smooth and thick. Pour into a glass and serve.

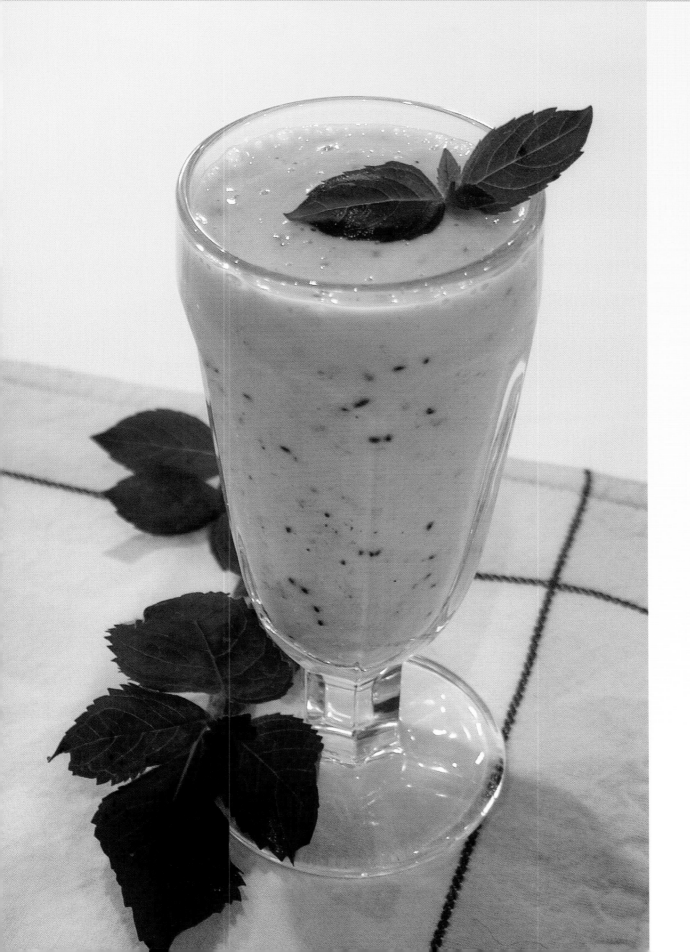

Dried Apricot and Blackberry Compote

Dried apricots are a concentrated source of useful nutrients, including beta carotene, potassium and iron. They contribute fibre and are generally considered to be an excellent health food. Select traditional dried apricots for this recipe, preferably organic, when trying to cleanse the system as the ready-to-eat type are treated with sulphur dioxide. Here they are combined with glorious juicy blackberries, traditionally considered to be a tonic for boosting the immune system and blood, and full of vitamins and minerals. Blackberries freeze well, so it is worth picking them in plentiful supplies when they are at their plump best and freezing them for winter salads. Spiked with a little mint, this compote is refreshing for breakfast or as a dessert.

Serves 4

225 g/8 oz/1 cup dried apricots
2 large mint sprigs
450 g/1 lb/2 cups blackberries
clear honey to serve (optional)

Place the mint and apricots in a bowl and pour in enough boiling water to cover them. Cover and leave to soak overnight.

Discard the mint and use scissors to cut the apricots in half or into thirds. Add the blackberries and mix the fruit very lightly. Chill for at least 30 minutes before serving, with honey to trickle over to taste.

Papaya and Grape Salad with Lime and Bay

Bay leaves are popular in savoury cooking but their delicate flavour is also excellent with fruit and in syrups. Bay is thought of as an antiseptic and an aid to digestion. Vitamin-rich papaya and lime are perfectly complemented by bay in this simple fruit salad that is the perfect follow-up to a cleansing main course or excellent for breakfast. Sweet, crisp grapes balance the smooth, slightly buttery papaya and tangy lime to perfection.

Serves 2

4 large bay leaves
1 tablespoon sugar
juice of 1 lime
175 g/6 oz sweet seedless green grapes
1 papaya, halved, seeded and cut into grape-size dice

Tear the bay leaves in half, crumpling them slightly, and place in a very small saucepan with the sugar and 4 tablespoons water. Bring to the boil and cook for about 30 seconds, until the bay leaves are aromatic. Remove from the heat and add the lime juice, then pour the mixture into a bowl.

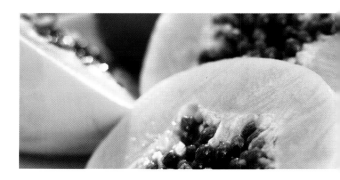

Add the grapes and papaya to the bowl and mix well. Cover and chill for several hours or overnight. Remove the pieces of bay leaf before serving the salad.

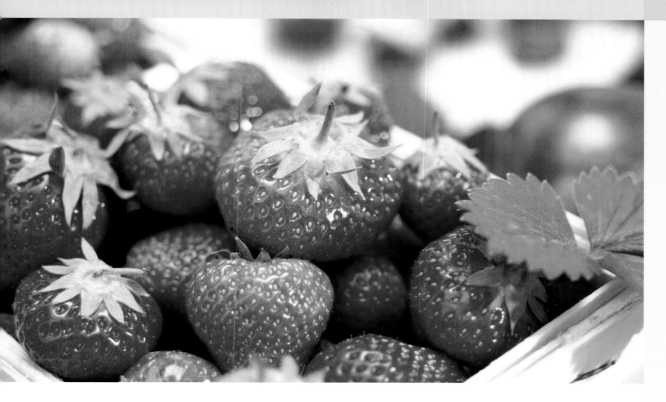

Orange-dressed Cherry and Strawberry Salad

This is a brilliant fruit salad for a detox diet. Cherries are renowned for encouraging the body to excrete toxins and strawberries are also purifying. Orange contributes additional vitamin C, an antioxidant that helps with the excretion of toxins. Luxuriate in this salad for breakfast or after any meal, or just indulge yourself with a fruity snack to boost your system. The rich, fruity mixture is spiked with juniper berries, which enrich the salad and make it more intriguing; they are also a cleansing spice that act as a diuretic and assist in the removal of toxins. Juniper is one of the spices used to flavour gin.

Serves 4

10 juniper berries
3 oranges
1 tablespoon honey
450 g/1 lb/2 cups cherries, pitted
450 g/1 lb/2 cups strawberries, hulled and halved

Crush the juniper berries finely in a mortar using a pestle, then place them in a small saucepan. Grate the rind and squeeze the juice from 1 orange, then add both to the juniper berries with the honey. Heat gently until boiling, then cover and remove from the heat. Leave to macerate for at least 1 hour – leave the mixture overnight if possible.

Cut the ends off the remaining oranges and cut off all the peel and pith in strips down the sides. Holding the fruit over a bowl to catch the juice, cut the segments from between the membranes and place them in the bowl. Add the cherries and strawberries, then pour in the juniper infusion, scraping every last drop from the pan. Lightly mix the salad, cover and chill before serving.

There are many ways of dealing with mental stress and the physically fraught pace of everyday life. It is sad that, for many, food and eating have become a focus for negative associations, when they can – and should – be enjoyable and calming. Not every meal provides an opportunity for a spot of soothing cooking but instead of dismissing food preparation as either a no-go area or a sophisticated hobby, it is a good idea to try and find a happy medium. For example, finding practical solutions to different types of meals is a good approach.

If everyday meals are a frantic hassle, the answer may be to plan ahead and maximize fridge and freezer resources for good eating. Instead of relying on highly processed bought meals, cooking favourite dishes in double quantities and freezing the excess for future use takes very little extra effort. (The trick is to reduce the forethought required by getting into the habit of cooking a little extra and having plenty of suitable containers or freezer bags handy, so that storing the surplus is not time consuming.) Stocking up on the right sort of frozen ingredients – plain fish and seafood, stir-fry poultry or meat, simple and mixed vegetables – is more conducive to a balanced diet than filling the cupboard, fridge or freezer with ready meal products. Canned fish, beans, pulses and tomatoes, along with passata and bottled marinated vegetables are useful storecupboard items for almost-instant meals. Focus on simple foods such as salad leaves and vegetables, breads, rice and pasta that take very little preparation and cooking. Remember eggs and cheese? They are nutritious, simple and quick to cook, as well as delicious to eat and very good for the nervous system when combined with a healthy balance of fruit and vegetables.

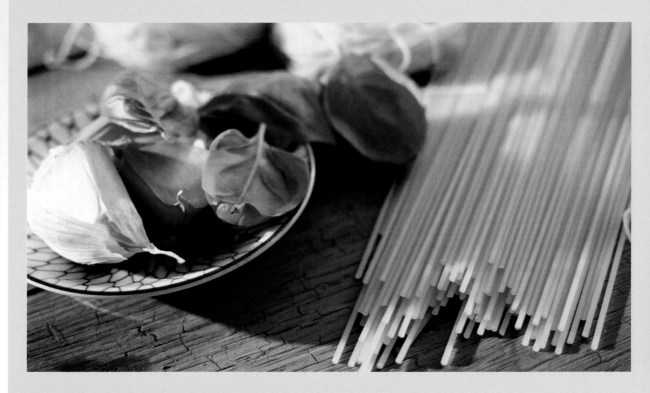

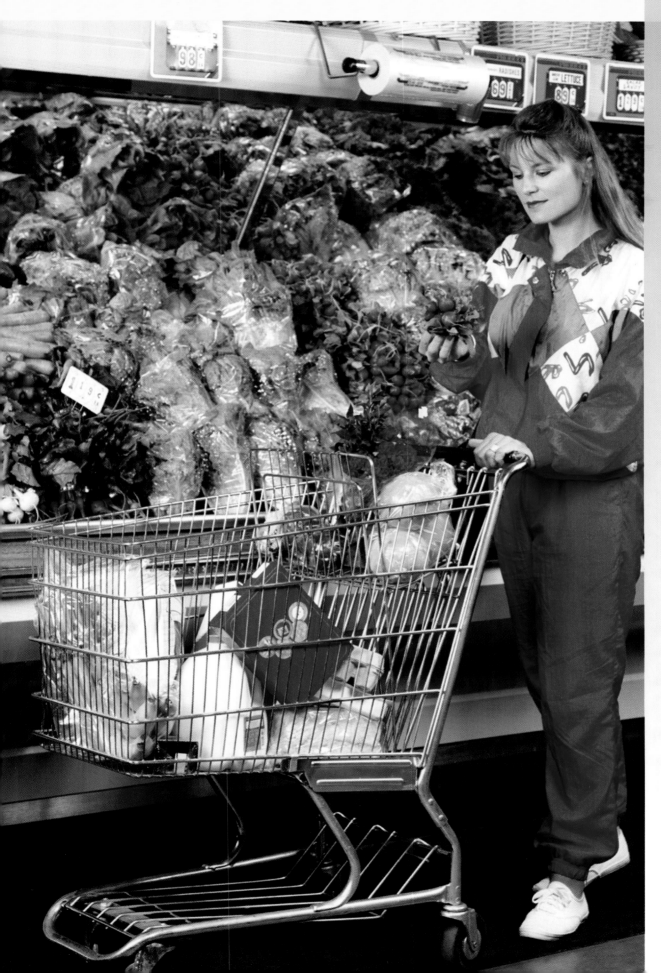

CALM AND SOOTHE

Physiologically, eating plenty of the right nutrients is important for the nervous system. B-group vitamins found in seafood, meat, eggs, yeast extract, dairy produce, green vegetables, cereals, pulses, seeds and dried fruit are calming. There should also be adequate supplies of the minerals selenium, zinc, manganese and potassium, and complex carbohydrate to prevent low blood sugar levels. Try to avoid the highs and lows associated with eating sugary foods that raise blood sugar levels without having adequate complex carbohydrate supplies to sustain the level. Complement this with calming camomile, lavender, marjoram, dill, and balancing herbs, such as mint and thyme.

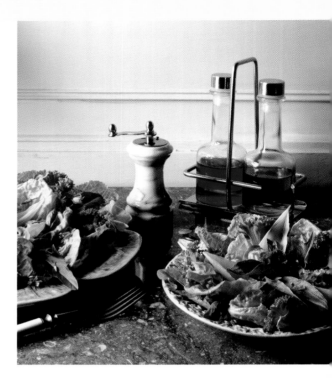

Most importantly, seek out the calming and soothing side of preparing food, cooking and eating. Think of the nurturing process and find the simple techniques and methods that you can relax into. For example, making time to prepare a simple salad and quietly slicing or cutting can be a very calming process. The choice of cooking methods is also important – whereas rapid stir-frying is lively and invigorating, stirring a smooth soup or a gently simmering risotto can be very calming. Simply standing over an aromatic pot of gently cooking ingredients can be relaxing. Making chutneys and preserves may be an area to explore, and baking can be very satisfying and relaxing. Making bread is a traditional form of relaxation, allowing time for reflection while kneading the dough – interesting that the repetitive physical process of kneading can almost be equated with taking gentle exercise. The smell, warmth and silky touch of the yeast dough are all calming.

Making simple dips, dressings and marinades can be very therapeutic. These are not last-minute recipes so their preparation does not have to be urgent or pressing. Salads and other raw dishes share this characteristic. Try to establish a small repertoire of dishes that you enjoy assembling and for which you do not have to refer to a recipe – make them your calming, soothing and escaping areas of cooking. Keep them simple when you do not want to think, or develop enjoyable ways of adapting and varying them for a more conscious kind of culinary relaxation.

The real message of this section is to discover simple enjoyment in food. Find your cooking therapy and learn how to escape into it.

Chickpea, Sundried Tomato and Basil Dip

Away from the bustle of entertaining or party-going, slowly sampling a soothing dip can be an excellent and healthy way to wind down at the end of a bad day. There is also something very calming about mashing and mixing this simple dip. Serve plenty of sesame breadsticks and little wholegrain crackers to dunk into the satisfying dip. Alternatively, serve the dip as a paté, with slices of wholemeal toast, or as a delicious filling for pitta bread or lengths of crusty baguette with salad.

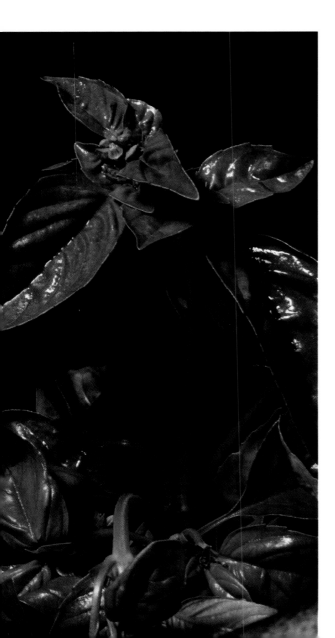

Serves 2

400 g/14 oz can chickpeas, drained
4 tablespoons tahini
6 sundried tomatoes packed in olive oil, drained
2 spring onions (scallions)
salt and pepper
4 large basil sprigs
squeeze of lemon juice

Turn the chickpeas into a bowl and crush them with a sturdy fork. Add the tahini and mash it into the chick peas to make a coarse paste.

Use kitchen scissors or a sharp knife for cutting up the remaining ingredients. Snip or dice the sundried tomatoes into small pieces and add them to the chickpea paste. Snip the spring onions into thin slices and mix them in with seasoning, to taste.

Finally, use scissors to shred the basil finely into the dip and add a squeeze of lemon juice. Then use a fork to mix in the basil and lemon. Taste for seasoning and lemon juice before transferring the dip to a serving bowl or two individual bowls.

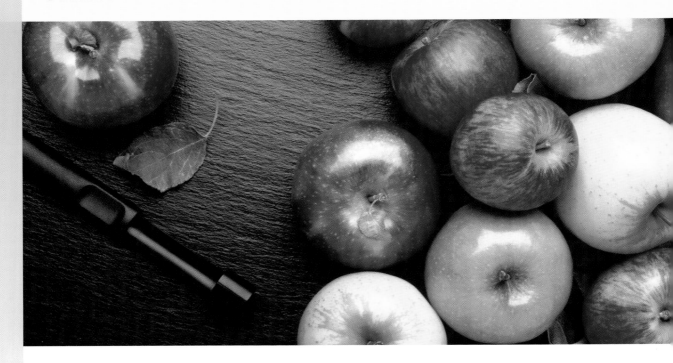

Warming Camomile, Carrot and Apple Soup

Straight camomile tea is something of an acquired taste but it is easy to benefit from the calming properties of the herb by using the tea instead of stock to make a soothing soup. Thickened with oats, this fruity soup provides all the right nutrients and perfect eating qualities to promote a wonderfully calm state of mind.

Serves 4

4 sachets camomile tea
2 tablespoons olive oil
1 onion, chopped
4 carrots, sliced
4 sage leaves
2 cooking apples, peeled, cored and roughly chopped
4 tablespoons rolled oats
600 ml/1 pint/2½ cups unsweetened apple juice

Place the sachets of tea in a heatproof measuring jug and pour in 600 ml/1 pint/2½ cups boiling water. Set aside to infuse.

Heat the olive oil in a saucepan and add the onion, carrots and sage. Stir to coat the vegetables in the oil, then cover the pan and cook gently for 15 minutes, until the onion has softened.

Discard the sachets from the camomile tea and pour it into the pan. Bring to the boil, then reduce the heat so that the soup simmers gently. Cover the pan and cook for 15 minutes. Add the apples and bring back to simmering point, then cook for a further 15 minutes. Sprinkle in the oats, cover and simmer for 10 minutes.

Purée the soup until smooth in a blender or food processor, then return it to the pan. Stir in the apple juice and reheat the soup, stirring continuously, until almost boiling. Ladle into bowls or large mugs and serve.

Creamy Almond Soup

This luscious soup is delicate and delicious. Nuts provide B vitamins and minerals that are important for a healthy nervous system. The smooth, scrumptious texture of this light soup is extremely soothing. Serve with slices of Marjoram and Dill Bread (page 97) as an accompaniment, for the benefit of these herbs' calming herbal qualities.

Serves 4

25 g/1 oz/2 tablespoons butter
175 g/6 oz/1½ cups blanched almonds
blade of mace
4 bay leaves
grated rind of ½ lemon
600 ml/1 pint/2½ cups chicken stock
300 ml/½ pint/1¼ cups milk
2 tablespoons rolled oats
salt and pepper
300 ml/½ pint/1¼ cups single (light) cream

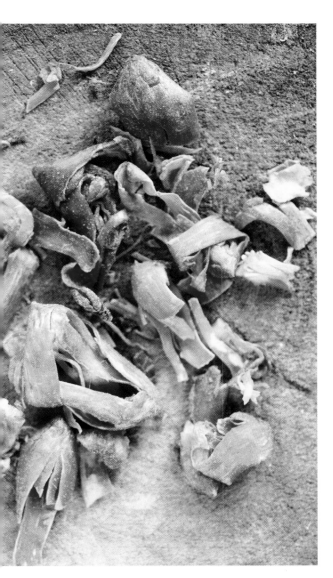

Melt the butter in a saucepan over low heat. Add the almonds and mace, and crumple the bay leaves into the pan. Cover and cook gently for 15 minutes, until the bay leaves and mace are aromatic.

Stir in the lemon rind, then pour in the stock and bring to the boil. Reduce the heat and cover the pan. Simmer the soup very gently for 15 minutes. Add the milk and rolled oats with a little salt and pepper. Bring to the boil, stirring, then immediately remove from the heat and leave to stand for 30 minutes.

Remove the bay leaves and mace from the soup and purée it in a food processor until smooth. Return the soup to the pan and heat it gently, stirring to just below boiling point. Stir in the cream and heat the soup gently without allowing it to simmer again. Ladle into bowls and serve at once.

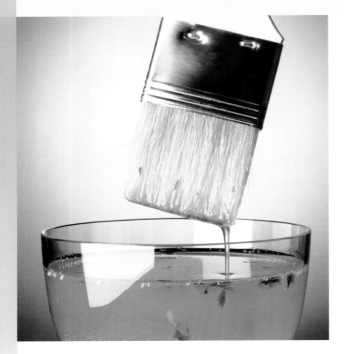

Marjoram, Rosemary and Mustard Marinade

This aromatic herb marinade brings together calming marjoram and rosemary, both thought to be especially helpful in relieving nervous tension, headaches and the associated nervous exhaustion. Use it with oily fish, particularly mackerel, poultry or meat. It is also excellent with small, whole, new or salad potatoes, either as a dressing for coating the freshly boiled vegetables, or as a marinade and basting liquid in which to roast them.

I tablespoon dried marjoram

2 teaspoons finely chopped dried rosemary

2 tablespoons wholegrain mustard

I tablespoon sugar

2 tablespoons cider vinegar

salt and pepper

6 tablespoons olive oil

Mix the marjoram, rosemary and mustard with the sugar, cider vinegar and seasoning. Whisk until the sugar has dissolved in the vinegar, then whisk in the oil. Use at once or store in a covered container in the fridge.

Marinated Mackerel

Place mackerel fillets skin sides up in a flame-proof dish large enough to hold them in just a single layer. Trickle the marinade evenly over them, then cover and chill for 1–3 hours. Preheat the grill (broiler) on the hottest setting. Turn the mackerel fillets so that they are skin side up and grill (broil) until browned. Turn and grill briefly on the second side, until the fish is just cooked. Serve at once.

Pork with Pumpkin

Cut lean, boneless pork into thin strips and place in a dish. Pour over the marinade, cover and chill for at least 1 hour or for as long as 24 hours. Prepare the peeled and seeded pumpkin, cutting it into 1 cm/½ in dice. Stir-fry the pumpkin in a little sunflower oil with plenty of chopped spring onions and crushed garlic until just tender – do not overcook the pumpkin, but leave it slightly crunchy. Use a slotted spoon to remove the pumpkin from the pan. Drain the meat, reserving the marinade, and stir-fry it until browned. Pour in the marinade and replace the pumpkin. Cook, stirring, for a few minutes. Serve with brown rice or couscous.

CALM AND SOOTHE

Lamb Kebabs

Marinate chunks of lean, boneless lamb (from the leg or fillet) overnight. Drain the pieces of meat, reserving the marinade, and thread them on to metal skewers with bay leaves, pickling onions and chunks of red and green pepper. Cook well away from the heat source under a preheated hot grill (broiler), turning often and brushing with the marinade. Serve with mixed wild and Camargue red rice, or couscous, and a spinach and watercress salad for a soothing meal rich in vitamins B and C, iron and carbohydrate.

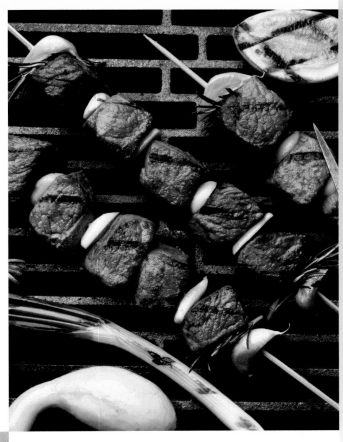

Potatoes and Pears

Use equal quantities of potatoes and pears. Cook some new or salad potatoes in their skins in boiling water for 10 minutes, until almost tender. Meanwhile, peel core and quarter firm pears and turn them in the marinade. Add the potatoes and mix well. Turn ingredients into an ovenproof dish just large enough to hold them in a single layer. Roast at 200°C/400°F/Gas 6 for about 45 minutes, until browned in places. Turn the ingredients occasionally so that they brown evenly. Serve the roasted potatoes and pears as an accompaniment for meat or poultry. Or try it on a bed of mixed leaves, topped with shreds of Parmesan and served with warm, crusty bread as a first course or light meal.

CALM AND SOOTHE

Hot Salmon Salad with Aromatic Walnut and Dolcelatte Pesto

Making this dish will lift your spirits and eating it will provide all the nourishment the body needs for physiological calming and soothing. The salad is packed with vitamins B12, A and D from the fish, vitamin C from the leafy base and a boost of B vitamins and minerals from the nut pesto. Cooking with warming, sunny basil is always a positive experience, so take the time to indulge in the sheer enjoyment of handling good ingredients in the simplest possible way when making this dish. Serve with plenty of closely textured country-style crusty bread to mop the delicious juices and provide a source of valuable carbohydrate.

Serves 2

100 g/4 oz/¾ cup walnuts
75 g/3 oz dolcelatte cheese
150 ml/¼ pint/⅔ cup olive oil
large handful of basil leaves and tender sprigs
salt and pepper
100 g/4 oz baby spinach leaves
100 g/4 oz watercress
100 g/4 oz lamb's lettuce
handful of chives, snipped
2 skinless boneless salmon steaks
salt and pepper
lemon wedges to serve

Finely grind the walnuts in a food processor. Cut the dolcelatte cheese into pieces and add to the nuts with about half the olive oil, then process until the mixture is a creamy paste. Add the basil and continue processing, pouring in the remaining oil with the motor running, to make a bright green, aromatic pesto. Taste the pesto and add seasoning if necessary.

Mix the spinach, watercress and lamb's lettuce and divide them between two large serving bowls or plates. Sprinkle with lots of snipped chives and dot a little pesto over the salad.

Have a warm plate ready for cutting up the cooked fish. Heat a heavy frying pan (skillet) or griddle and grease it lightly with a little olive oil. Add the salmon steaks and cook for 3–4 minutes on each side, until lightly browned and cooked through. The flesh should flake easily but still be moist and succulent.

Transfer the salmon steaks to the warm plate and cut them into small chunks. Distribute these over the salads and top with more pesto. Add the lemon wedges and serve at once, offering the remaining pesto separately.

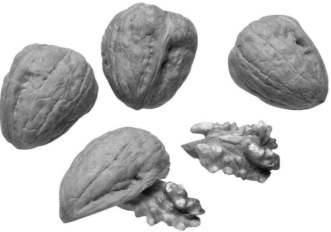

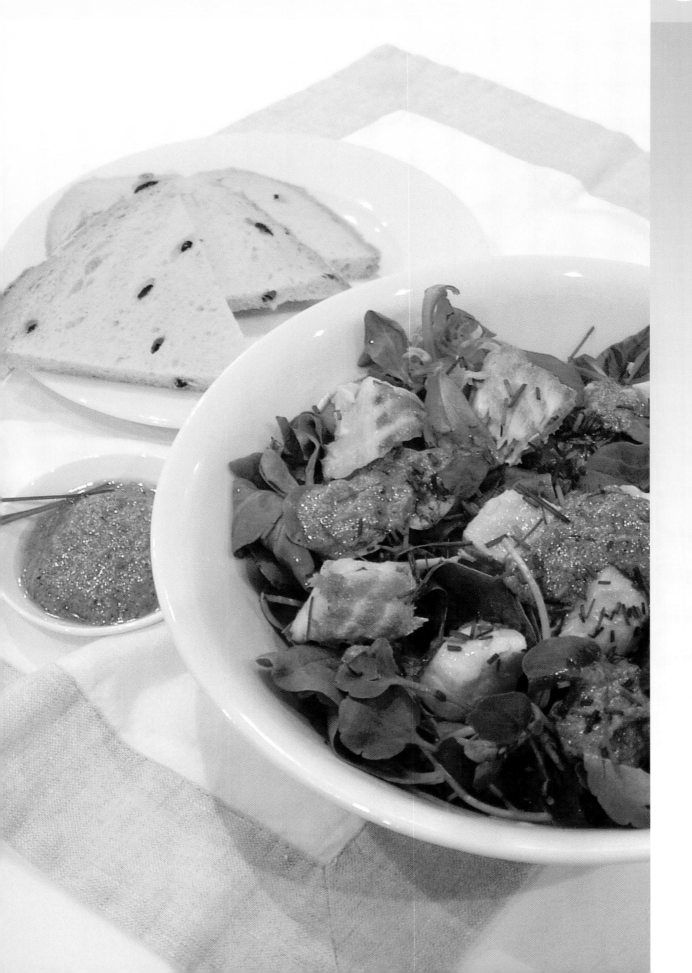

CALM AND SOOTHE

Cod on Herb-drenched Croûtes with Roasted Peppers and Pine Nuts

Any firm white fish tastes delicious cooked this way as, indeed, do the oily fish, such as tuna or salmon. The important features of this dish are the simplicity of preparation and the sense of fulfilment that cooking it can bring, combined with the nutritional benefits of eating a diet rich in vitamins and minerals that help to boost the nervous system. Thyme is one of those herbs that is thought of as bringing a balance – providing a mix of calming and uplifting influences to soothe and encourage sleep but also to stimulate the appetite and lift the spirits. Here it is combined with calming dill on fabulous herb-topped croûtes. Select sturdy bread for the croûtes – ideally home-made – so that they absorb all the wonderful juices and flavours of the other ingredients.

Serves 2

3 tablespoons olive oil
2 thick slices seeded wholemeal bread, crusts removed
2 large red (bell) peppers, seeded and cut into thin strips
1 leek, thinly sliced
salt and pepper
handful each of thyme and dill sprigs
2 large, thick portions cod fillet, skinned
2 tablespoons pine nuts

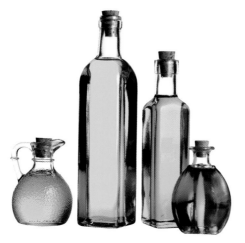

Preheat the oven to 200°C/400°F/Gas 6. Brush about a third of the oil over the bread, covering the slices lightly on both sides. Heat a large, heavy frying pan (skillet)and brown the bread on both sides, then transfer the slices to a large, shallow ovenproof dish.

Add about half the remaining oil to the pan. Swirl it around, then add the pepper slices and turn them over and over for a few seconds over high heat to soften them and lightly brown them in places. Use a fish slice to remove them from the pan and set aside on a plate.

Add the leeks to the oil and juices in the pan. Season them well and reduce the heat, then cook for about 10 minutes, stirring often, until they are softened and reduced. Remove the pan from the heat.

Pick all the leaves off the thyme and discard any tough stalks from the dill, then divide the prepared herbs between the bread slices, piling up the leaves and tender sprigs. Arrange about half the peppers and half the leeks on top of the herbs, then place a portion of cod on each piece of bread. Spoon more leeks and peppers on top of the fish and arrange any remaining vegetables around the croûtes in the dish, spooning any juices over the fish.

Sprinkle the pine nuts over the fish croûtes and drizzle the remaining oil over the top. Bake for about 30 minutes, until the topping on the fish is browned and the fish flakes easily. Serve at once.

Saffron Risotto with Pan-fried Oregano Prawns

Prawns provide vitamin B12 and selenium, both useful nutrients for a healthy nervous system. Served with aromatic herbs on a creamy risotto, they make a splendid meal. The dish is also brilliant for the fact that it is simple to prepare, without any need for lengthy preparation or complicated techniques. The minimum of chopping is followed by gentle stirring, just the method for inducing a sense of calm. So take time out to encourage the rice towards that tender creamy consistency that is so soothing to eat.

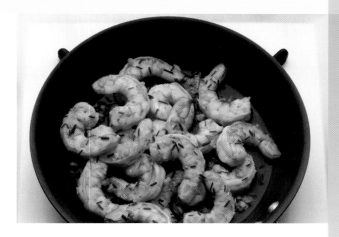

Serves 2

225 g/8 oz raw peeled tiger prawns
1 teaspoon dried oregano
1 garlic clove, crushed
grated rind of 1 lemon and juice of ½ lemon
2 tablespoons olive oil
100 g/4 oz rocket
large handful of dill sprigs, tough stalks discarded

Saffron Risotto

½ teaspoon saffron strands
450 ml/¾ pint/2 cups hot chicken stock
2 tablespoons olive oil
1 small onion, finely chopped
2 bay leaves
salt and pepper
225 g/8 oz/1 cup risotto rice
300 ml/½ pint/1¼ cups dry white wine
4 tablespoons freshly grated Parmesan cheese

Place the prawns in a bowl. Add the oregano, garlic and lemon rind. Mix well and set aside.

For the risotto, pound the saffron strands to a powder in a mortar and add a couple of spoonfuls of the hot stock to dissolve the powder, then set aside. Heat the olive oil in a heavy saucepan. Add the onion and bay leaves with salt and pepper, stir well and cover the pan. Cook gently for 10 minutes, then uncover the pan and cook gently for a further 5 minutes, until the onion is softened but not browned.

Add the rice to the onion and stir for 2–3 minutes, until the grains are coated with the oil in the pan. Pour in about half the stock and bring to the boil, then reduce the heat and allow the rice to simmer gently, stirring occasionally. Gradually add the remaining stock as the rice absorbs the liquid. Then pour in the wine and bring it to the boil. Reduce the heat and simmer gently again, stirring occasionally, until the liquid is absorbed. Sprinkle the saffron liquid over the risotto, stir lightly and cover the pan, then remove it from the heat and set aside.

Heat the olive oil for the prawns in a frying pan (skillet). Add the prawns and cook them for 2–3 minutes on each side, until they are pink and tender. Do not overcook them or they will shrivel and become tough. Remove the pan from the heat and add seasoning to taste with the lemon juice.

Divide the risotto among two bowls. Stir the rocket and dill into the prawns and immediately spoon them on to the risotto. Serve at once.

CALM AND SOOTHE

Escalopes of Pork with Salad Potato, Broccoli and Sage Gratin

A combination of soothing flavours, satisfying ingredients and nutrients to promote a healthy nervous system make this an excellent recipe for inducing calm. Also, from the practical point of view, the dish involves little more than lightly boiling and assembling ingredients to make a tempting and complete meal. Add a good mixed leafy salad with thinly sliced green pepper to complement this main dish, or have a hearty fruit salad to follow.

Serves 2

350 g/12 oz salad potatoes, sliced
350 g/12 oz small broccoli florets
a little olive oil
2 large pork escalopes
2 large sage sprigs
bunch of spring onions (scallions), sliced
salt and pepper
4 tablespoons fresh breadcrumbs
2 tablespoons freshly grated Parmesan cheese
150 g/5 oz/1 cup mozzarella cheese, diced

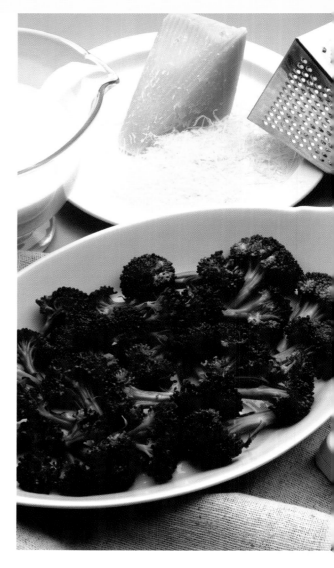

Preheat the oven to 180°C/350°F/ Gas 4. Place the potatoes in a saucepan and pour in boiling water to cover. Bring to the boil, then reduce the heat and simmer gently for 7–10 minutes, until the potatoes are tender.

Use a draining spoon to remove the potatoes from the pan and transfer them to a plate. Add the broccoli to the water remaining in the pan and bring back to the boil. Cook for 1 minute, then drain and rinse under cold water. Drain well.

Grease a large ovenproof dish with a little olive oil and lay the pork escalopes in it. Pick the sage leaves off their stalks and sprinkle them over the pork. Add the spring onions, spreading them out evenly over the pork, then season to taste. Arrange the potatoes over the pork and top with the broccoli, allowing the vegetables to overlap the escalopes if there is not enough room on top.

Mix the breadcrumbs, Parmesan and mozzarella cheese and spoon this mixture evenly over the vegetables. Place the gratin in the oven and cook for about 45 minutes, until the pork is cooked, the dish is aromatic with sage and well browned and crisp on top. Serve at once.

CALM AND SOOTHE

Baked Eggs with Spinach and Potatoes

Eggs and vegetables are good foods for calming and soothing, especially when prepared simply but in a slightly special way. Baked in large individual dishes, these require virtually no last-minute attention – the vegetable bases can be assembled ready for the eggs to be added when you are ready to put supper in the oven. Trickled with cream and seasoned with a hint of nutmeg, these make a deliciously soothing supper when served with thinly sliced wholemeal bread.

Serves 2

350 g/12 oz potatoes, diced
salt and pepper
450 g/1 lb baby spinach
25 g/1 oz/2 tablespoons butter
1 teaspoon dried marjoram
4 eggs
4 tablespoons single (light) or double (heavy) cream, or milk
a little freshly grated nutmeg

Preheat the oven to 180°C/350°F/Gas 4. Cook the potatoes in boiling salted water for 7–10 minutes, until tender, then drain well. Rinse the spinach and place it in the saucepan. Cover and cook over medium heat, shaking the pan often, for about 5 minutes, until the spinach is greatly reduced in volume. Drain thoroughly.

Grease two individual ovenproof dishes or one larger dish with a little of the butter. Add the spinach and sprinkle with the marjoram, then top with the potatoes. Use a dessertspoon to shuffle neat holes in the spinach and potatoes to hold the eggs.

Crack an egg into each hole in the vegetables. Dot the remaining butter over the vegetables and eggs, then trickle the cream over the eggs. Sprinkle with a little nutmeg and bake for 10–15 minutes, until the eggs are set to taste. Serve at once.

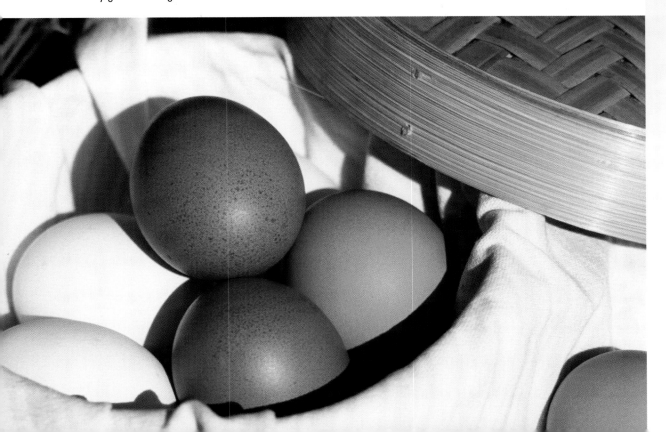

CALM AND SOOTHE

Couscous with Egg and Anchovy Salad

When the world feels like one big hassle take refuge in a little simple food preparation. Instant couscous is effortless and the rest of this dish needs the very minimum of attention. To make a single portion, prepare half the quantities – the extra anchovies will keep in a covered container in the fridge for 1–2 days.

Serves 2

2 tablespoons cumin seeds
grated rind and juice of 1 lime
100 g/4 oz couscous
2 Little Gem lettuce hearts, shredded
225 g/8 oz fine green beans, cooked
2 spring onions (scallions), thinly sliced
50 g/2 oz can anchovies
10–12 black olives, sliced
10 cherry tomatoes, halved
4 eggs, hard boiled and roughly chopped

Roast the cumin seeds in a small, heavy pan over low heat until they are aromatic, shaking the pan often. Immediately transfer them to a small heatproof bowl and add the couscous and lime rind. Pour in just enough freshly boiling water to cover the couscous, and stir. Cover the bowl with cling film (saran wrap). Set aside for 15–20 minutes, until the water is all absorbed and the couscous is tender.

Meanwhile, mix the lettuce and beans with the spring onions and divide among two large salad bowls or plates. Drain the oil from the anchovies into a bowl. Chop the anchovies or snip them into the bowl using kitchen scissors. Add the lime juice and mix well. Stir in the olives and tomatoes. Then add the eggs and mix lightly. Divide the couscous among the bowls, mounding it slightly, and spoon the egg and anchovy salad over.

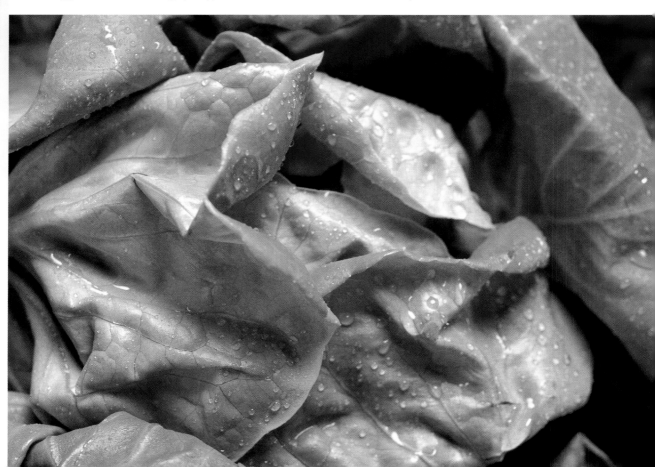

Simple Carrot, Apricot and Feta Salad

The very idea of preparing and the simple method of creating this salad is intended as a soothing, healing process. Take time out to nurture yourself and those for whom you are cooking and bring them a message of caring and sharing with all the good ingredients this salad offers. Warming marjoram, marinated with mellow olive oil and subtly citric orange makes a fabulous dressing for the crisp carrots and punchy feta with tangy-sweet apricots.

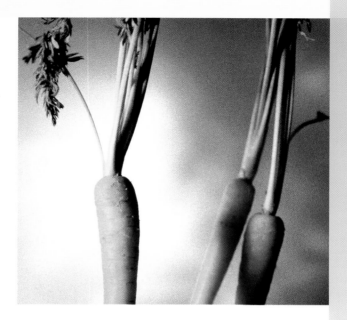

Serves 2-4

4 large marjoram sprigs or 1 teaspoon dried marjoram
juice of 1 orange
3 tablespoons good extra virgin olive oil
handful of chives
175 g/6 oz/1 cup ready-to-eat dried apricots
200 g/7 oz/1 cup feta cheese
8 large carrots

Pick the leaves off the marjoram and place them in a small saucepan, alternatively place the dried marjoram in the pan. Add the orange juice and bring to the boil over low heat, until the marjoram is aromatic. Remove from the heat, and pour into a salad bowl. Add the olive oil and chives and set aside.

Use kitchen scissors to snip the apricots into slices. Alternatively, slice them with a knife. Then add them to the dressing in the bowl. Crumble the cheese by hand into the bowl. Stir the apricots and cheese gently with the dressing. Cover and set aside.

Prepare a large bowl of iced water. Use a vegetable peeler to prepare the carrots. Wash and peel them, leaving the ends in place. Peel off ribbons of carrot and add them to the

bowl of water. Curve the strips down into the carrots as you peel them off so that they tend to curl. Begin at one end of the carrot, so that there is enough space for peeling out a second curve of strips from further down. You will be left with the ends and the edge of carrot with two deep curves – trim off the ends and use this in other recipes calling for diced or chopped carrot, or simply eat it up as a snack.

You have two options at this point: to drain the carrots and dry them in a salad spinner or leave the strips to soak in the water until they curl. Leave them for an hour and they will be lightly curled and the longer you leave them the more wonderfully curly they become. After 2–3 hours, they form fabulous carrot rings that curl in the dressing picking up just enough of it to taste amazing.

Toss the carrots into the salad at the last minute and serve immediately. If they are allowed to stand for any length of time they wilt and become straight – they are still edible but not as much fun and they lose the ability to pick up the perfect amount of dressing, becoming drenched rather than showered by the delicious juices.

CALM AND SOOTHE

Seeded Milk Bread

Breadmaking is so soothing. Gently turning, pressing and kneading the warm soft dough is a calming and therapeutic process. The waiting and proving is cut out when using modern, easy-blend yeast that needs just the one rising. So it is easy to indulge in the enjoyable dough handling without having to wait and go back to the risen dough to knock it back and shape it – a blessing for today's busy lifestyle. Rather than thinking in terms of kneading out your frustrations on the dough, make this a positive process and see it as a gentle exercise to restore peace of mind, taking time out to relax. And at the end of the baking session there is wonderful aromatic bread packed with seeds that contribute useful B vitamins to the wholemeal bread.

Makes 2 loaves

good handful each of sunflower and pumpkin seeds
4 tablespoons sesame seeds
2 tablespoons fennel seeds
2 tablespoons linseeds (optional)
2 tablespoons mustard seeds (optional)
I tablespoons caraway seeds (optional)
450 g/I lb/4 cups strong wholemeal flour
I sachet fast-action easy-blend yeast
I teaspoon salt
I teaspoon dried oregano
I teaspoon sugar
250 ml/8 fl oz/I cup hand-hot milk
2 tablespoons olive oil

Roast the sunflower and pumpkin seeds separately in a small, heavy pan for a few minutes over moderated heat until they are beginning to brown. Shake the pan often and tip the seeds out into a large bowl as soon as they are brown to prevent them from overcooking. Then roast the fennel seeds, linseeds, mustard and caraway seeds separately in the same way, tipping them all into the bowl as soon as they are ready.

Add the flour to the bowl. Stir in the yeast, salt, oregano and sugar. Make a well in the middle of the dry ingredients and pour in the milk. Add the olive oil and gradually incorporate the flour mixture to make a firm dough. Turn the dough out on to a lightly floured surface and knead it for about 10 minutes, until it is smooth and elastic.

Divide the dough in half and shape it into two slightly elongated loaves. Place these on greased baking sheets and cover them loosely with oiled cling film (saran wrap) or clean tea towels. Leave in a warm place until doubled in size.

Preheat the oven to 220°C/425°F/Gas 7. Brush the tops of the loaves with warm water and make three diagonal slits across each one.

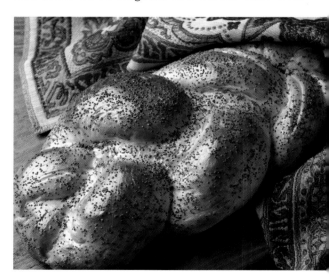

Bake for about 40 minutes, until the bread is crusty and brown. Cool on a wire rack.

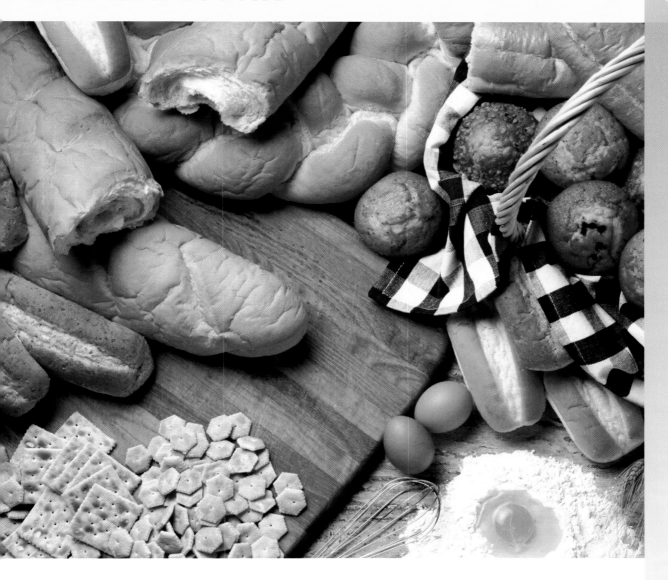

Flavouring Bread Dough

Herbs are especially good in bread dough, either singly or mixed.

Marjoram and Dill Bread: omit the oregano – the seeds can be retained or omitted as preferred. Finely chop a large bunch of fresh dill and add to the flour mixture with 1 tablespoon dried marjoram.

Spring Onion and Sage Bread: finely chop a bunch of spring onions and a handful of fresh sage leaves. Omit the oregano and seeds, and add the spring onions and sage instead.

Using a Bread Maker Machine

The sort of bread machines that mix and knead ingredients, then churn out finished loaves are brilliant and the result is still a kitchen – or house – filled with the comforting aroma of freshly baked bread. The bread itself is also delicious and wholesome. Follow the manufacturer's instructions for multigrain or wholemeal bread, adding the mixture of seeds used above. When adapting recipes for bread machines, you have to experiment – the golden rule is not to overload the machine, so make a half quantity if you are worried about using too great a weight of ingredients.

Blackcurrant and Apricot Bran Muffins

These muffins are have a high fibre content and a modest amount of sugar. They provide the body with complex carbohydrate as a slow-release source of energy, helping to keep blood sugar levels stable. The blackcurrants make a valuable contribution of vitamin C and the dried apricots provide iron, potassium and beta carotene.

Makes 12

225 g/8 oz/2 cups wholemeal flour
4 tablespoons bran
1 tablespoon baking powder
50 g/2 oz/⅓ cup soft (light) brown sugar
100 g/4 oz/½ cup ready-to-eat dried apricots, chopped
175 g/6 oz/¾ cup fresh or frozen blackcurrants
1 egg
2 tablespoons sunflower oil
100 ml/7 fl oz/½ cup milk

Preheat the oven to 200°C/400°F/Gas 6 and grease 12 large, muffin pans. Mix the flour, bran, baking powder and sugar in a bowl. Make a well in the middle of the dry ingredients and add the apricots and blackcurrants.

Beat the egg with the sunflower oil and milk, then pour the mixture over the fruit in the middle of the bowl. Stir the dry ingredients into the fruit and liquid, taking care not to crush the blackcurrants. The ingredients should be just mixed, not overworked.

Divide the mixture among the prepared tins and bake for 15–20 minutes, until the muffins are well risen, cracked on top and springy to the touch. Leave them to cool in the tins for a few minutes, until they are firm enough to be transferred to a wire rack and left to cool. The muffins taste wonderful warm.

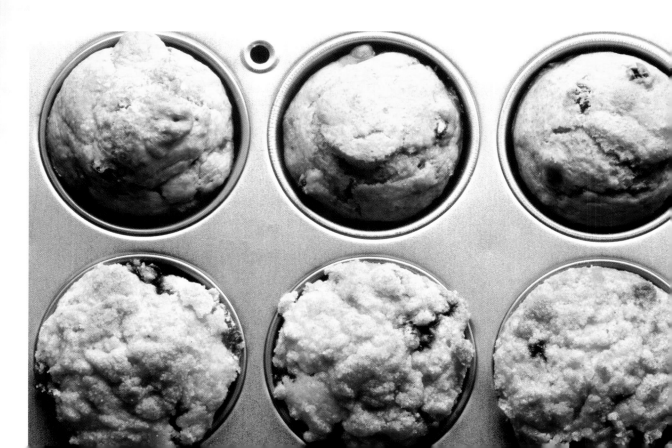

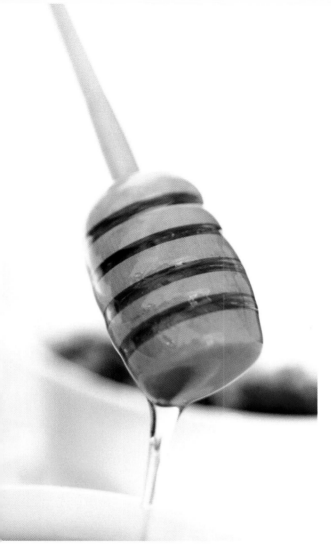

Banana and Blackcurrant Iced Yogurt

This is a whiz of a dessert and especially good for introducing oodles of vitamin C to wintry days. Freeze blackcurrants during the summer months to ensure you have a plentiful supply.

Serves 4

350 g/12 oz/2 cups frozen blackcurrants
2 tablespoons clear honey (or to taste)
600 ml/1 pint/2½ cups Greek-style yogurt
2 bananas

Whiz the frozen blackcurrants to a coarse purée in a food processor or blender with the honey. Add the yogurt and whiz again to make a thick, iced slush.

Peel and slice the bananas, then place in a bowl. Turn the iced yogurt mixture into the bowl and fold it with the bananas. Taste for sweetness, adding extra honey, if liked. Spoon into bowls and serve at once.

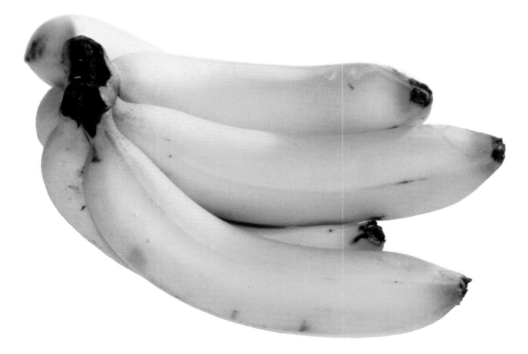

CALM AND SOOTHE

Lavender Zabaglione

Lavender is renowned for its calming properties. It is also scented and summery in this rich, warm and creamy dessert. Relax into the process of gently whisking and foaming the eggs to pale perfection, then indulge in the soothing results.

Serves 4

100 ml/4 fl oz/½ cup sweet white wine
flowers from 4 lavender sprigs
75 g/3 oz/3 tablespoons sugar
4 egg yolks
sponge fingers to serve

Pour the wine into a small saucepan and add the lavender. Heat gently until just simmering, stirring all the time, then cover and set aside to cool completely. Leave the lavender and wine to infuse for several hours or overnight, if possible.

Place the sugar in a large heatproof bowl and add the egg yolks. Strain the lavender-infused wine over the yolks and place the bowl over a saucepan of barely simmering water. Do not allow the water to overheat or reach simmering point or this may curdle the eggs.

Whisk the mixture using an electric whisk (beater) until it is pale, thick and creamy. The zabaglione should be light and foamy. Pour it into four warmed, tall glasses and serve at once, with sponge fingers for dipping.

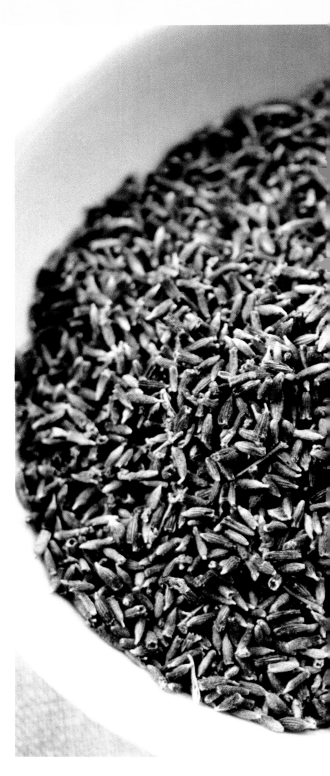

Apple, Rosemary and Camomile Tea

Camomile is the classic soothing and calming herb for making tea but rosemary is also known for helping to stimulate the nervous system and ease headaches. This is the perfect drink if you find the rather 'green' flavour of neat camomile challenging. To benefit from soothing drinks, make a point of taking time out to sip them – this may be while alone or in a few minutes of shared relaxation with your partner or family. Sitting comfortably, in a warm, calm and relaxing environment for just 5 minutes is a good practice for quelling the pace and finding a few minutes' peace of mind and body.

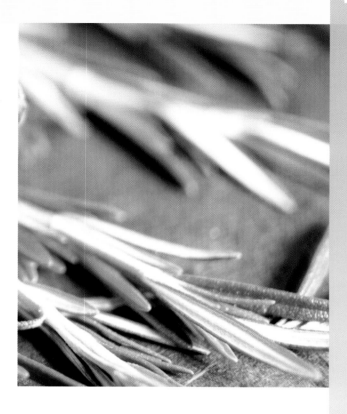

Serves 1

1 fresh rosemary sprig
1 sachet camomile tea
about 150 ml/¼ pint/⅔ cup unsweetened apple juice

Place the rosemary in a cup or glass and pour in boiling water to half fill the glass. Stir well, then add the camomile tea and leave to infuse for 3 minutes. Remove the sachet, squeezing it well, but leave the rosemary in the tea. Top up with the apple juice and a little extra boiling water, if liked.

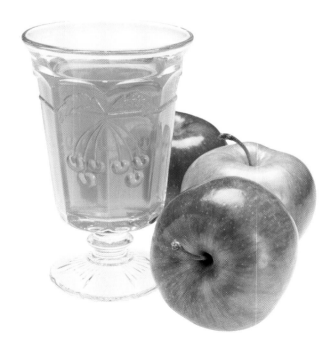

Physically, a balanced diet is essential for energy and that means plenty of fresh fruit and vegetables with a good supply of complex carbohydrate, daily amounts of good quality protein and all the minerals and vitamins necessary to keep the body in tip-top condition. Variety in the choice of ingredients, types of dishes and cooking methods is the key to maintaining a healthy diet in the long term.

In addition to the nutritional requirements, a positive outlook promotes a vital approach to food and eating. Just as every well-balanced activity in life has energetic highs to complement a gentler side, so cooking should include vigorous and vital dishes as well as calming, soothing, comforting and refreshing recipes. Discovering the contrasting colours, textures and flavours of foods, and the ways in which they can be combined, brings a whole new vitality to cooking and eating. This is all about inspiration and enthusiasm – but that does not mean creating a new meal every day. The very thought of cooking a favourite dish or familiar combination of ingredients can be enlivening.

Quick cooking methods and a 'kitchen active' approach are good to remember for the vigour they can introduce to your culinary life. Lighten up and try to find an open-minded approach to food – explore the idea of using different flavours with familiar techniques or in old favourite recipes. And share food and cooking with others, making it a caring process that can be humorous or full of fun as well as gentle.

The selection of recipes in this chapter reflects the fun that can be found in cooking and eating. Eclectic cooking styles and culinary combinations are the key features but nothing is complicated or difficult. On the contrary, combined with an appreciation of textures, colours, herbs and spices that stimulate, the recipes are intended to encourage a fresh approach that supports good basic nutrition in simple, lively cooking.

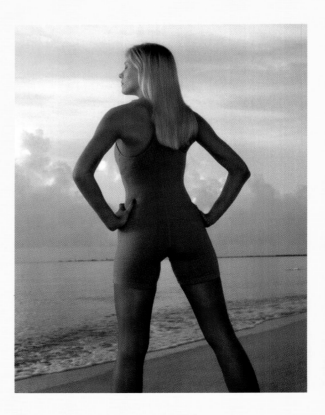

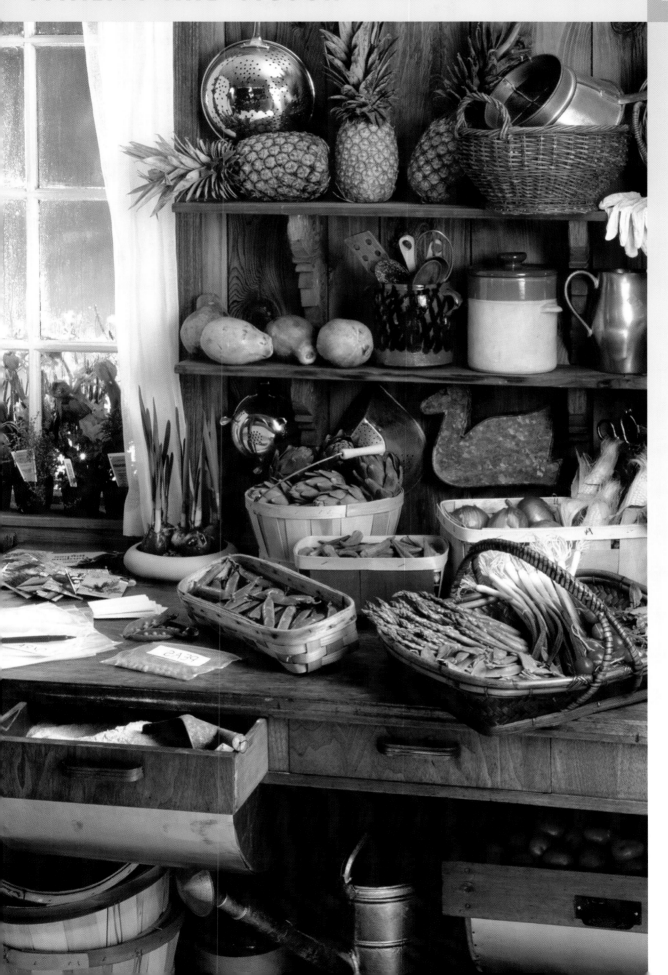

Slightly Spicy Red Vegetable Soup

This light soup is refreshing with ginger and cardamom, and packed with the beta carotene and phytochemical goodness of red vegetables. Simmering and stirring it up makes you feel good and it tastes terrific. It is the ideal winter soup for imparting energy and vitality – instead of a smooth texture to blanket out the world, the lively colours and open texture of vegetables in warming broth bring a real sparkle to the meal. Serve warm, crusty bread as an accompaniment. The soup will keep well in the fridge for 2–3 days, or it also freezes well for at least 3 months. So enjoy making a big pot of broth because it will provide instant meals at a later date.

Serves 8

6 green cardamoms
2 tablespoons sunflower oil
2 onions, finely chopped
25 g/1 oz fresh root ginger, peeled and finely chopped
coarsely grated zest of ½ large orange
3 red (bell) peppers, seeded and diced
350 g/12 oz carrots, diced
½ swede (rutabaga), 500–600 g/1lb 2oz–1lb 5oz, diced
1 large potato, diced
salt and pepper
1.5 litres/2¾ pints/7 cups turkey, chicken or vegetable stock

Slit the papery cardamoms and scrape out the black seeds into a mortar, then crush them with a pestle. Heat the oil in a large saucepan and add the onions, crushed cardamoms, ginger, orange zest and peppers. Cook, stirring, for about 10 minutes, until the onions are softened slightly.

Add the carrots, swede and potato. Sprinkle in a little seasoning and stir for a few seconds. Pour in the stock – the vegetables should be well covered – and bring to the boil. Immediately the soup boils, reduce the heat so that it just bubbles and cover the pan. Simmer the soup gently for 30 minutes, until the diced vegetables are tender but not falling. Taste the soup for seasoning – it should be sweet and delicate

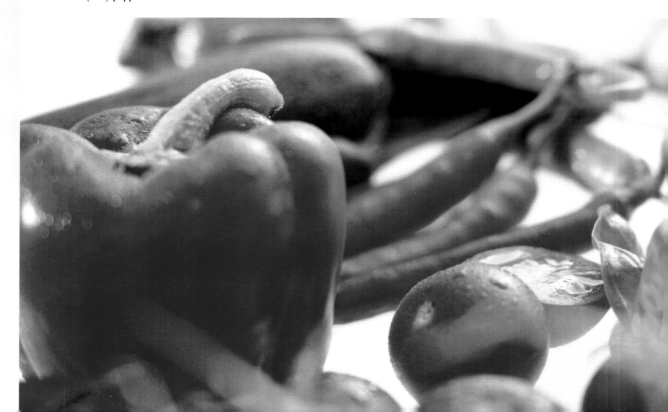

Green Vegetable Soup

Pepped with garlic and warming, invigorating nutmeg, then topped with a crunchy mixture of croûtons and chorizo on some shreds of basil, this soup tastes terrific. It is excellent for times when you are snowed under with a thousand things to do and have not had time to shop for fresh vegetables because it relies on frozen ingredients – and they are the positive type that bring plenty of vitamins to the diet. While the hot soup is perfect for winter, for a cool summer's day you may like to cool and chill the soup, then serve it swirled with yogurt or single (light) cream and with ice cubes floating in it, rather than croûtons and chorizo.

Serves 4

small knob of butter
1 tablespoon olive oil, plus extra for cooking croûtons
2 bay leaves
1 onion, chopped
2 large garlic cloves, crushed
1 small carrot, diced
1 large potato, diced
900 ml/1½ pints/3¾ cups ham or chicken stock
salt and pepper
225 g/8 oz/1¾ cups frozen petits pois
100 g/4 oz/1 cup frozen spinach
freshly grated nutmeg

Garnish
75 g/3 oz/2 tablespoons chorizo, finely diced
2 thick slices good wholemeal bread
handful of tender basil sprigs (optional)

Heat the butter and oil together in a large saucepan over medium heat until the butter melts. Add the bay leaves, onion, garlic and carrot, and cook, stirring for 2–3 minutes, until the vegetables are evenly coated in oil and butter. Cover the pan and cook the vegetables for 5 minutes.

Stir in the potato and pour in the stock. Add a little salt and pepper. Bring to the boil, reduce the heat and cover the pan, then simmer for 10 minutes.

Add the petits pois, bring the soup back to the boil and reduce the heat again, then cover and simmer for a further 5 minutes. Finally, stir in the spinach and bring back to the boil. Reduce the heat and simmer, covered, for 5 minutes. By this time the peas should be well cooked and the potatoes soft and falling.

Prepare the garnish while the soup is cooking. Dry fry the chorizo in a heavy pan until the fat runs and the dice are very small and well cooked. Use a draining spoon to remove the chorizo from the pan, then add a little olive oil to the fat from the chorizo, and toss in the cubes of bread (these can be quite chunky). Fry the croûtons, stirring and turning them frequently, until crisp and brown. Mix with the chorizo and set aside.

Cool the soup slightly and discard the bay leaves before puréeing it until smooth in a blender or using a hand-held blender. Return the soup to the pan, if necessary, taste for seasoning and add a little nutmeg. Reheat the soup, if necessary, stirring all the time, and ladle it into large bowls. Finely shred the basil with scissors, then sprinkle over the soup. Top with croûtons and chorizo and serve immediately.

Ginger-laced Fruity Cucumber Soup

Gloriously scented mango brings a burst of flavour and colour to cooling and refreshing cucumber in this chilled soup. Enlivening ginger combines with beta carotene and vitamin C from the mango for a helpful boost to wellbeing. Swirled with yogurt and honey before serving, the soup makes a fabulous summery lunch with bran muffins for the complex carbohydrate that helps to provide sustained energy. Chill the cucumber, mangoes, lemon and yogurt in advance so that the soup can be served freshly whizzed.

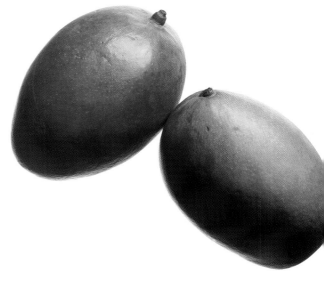

Serves 4

25 g/1 oz fresh root ginger, peeled and chopped
1 cucumber, cut into chunks
2 ripe mangoes, peeled, stoned (pitted) and cut into chunks
150 ml/¼ pint/⅔ cup water
juice of 1 lemon
300 ml/½ pint/1 cup plain yogurt
about 2 tablespoons clear honey
4 tablespoons chopped lemon balm (optional)

Purée the ginger with the cucumber until smooth in a blender or food processor. Add the mangoes and purée again until smooth. Then add the water and lemon juice and whiz the soup again until smooth.

Divide the soup among four bowls. Stir the yogurt until smooth and swirl it on top of the soup. Trickle with honey and sprinkle with lemon balm (if using). Serve immediately.

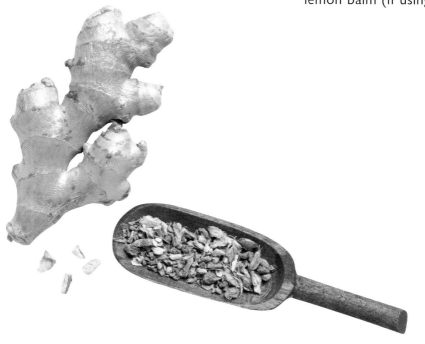

Golden Stir-fried Fish

A diet full of fruit and vegetables, and full of all the other essential nutrients in the right proportion, promotes vitality and energy. As well bright green beans and delicious spinach, this stir-fry has plenty of onions and garlic, along with stimulating turmeric. Adding spring onions (scallions) and lemon rind at the end of cooking brings an incredibly fresh and lively flavour to the dish, making it zingy and invigorating. Serve it with a modest portion of Chinese egg noodles or Japanese soba noodles – made from buckwheat flour – for an energizing main meal.

Serves 2

2 teaspoons ground turmeric

grated rind and juice of 1 lemon

salt and pepper

350 g/12 oz thick white fish fillet, skinned and cut into chunks

2 tablespoons sunflower oil

25 g/1 oz fresh root ginger, peeled and chopped

1 large onion, halved and thinly sliced

4 garlic cloves, thinly sliced

225 g/8 oz fine green beans

225 g/8 oz baby spinach leaves

4 spring onions (scallions), thinly sliced

Mix the turmeric, lemon juice and salt and pepper in a bowl. Add the fish and turn the pieces in the turmeric mixture to coat them evenly. Set aside.

Heat the oil in a large frying pan (skillet) or wok. Add the ginger, onion and garlic and stir-fry until the onion is softened and the garlic and ginger are aromatic. Add the green beans and continue to stir-fry until they are slightly tender, but still crisp. Use a draining spoon to remove the vegetables from the pan and set aside.

Add the fish, scraping in all the turmeric juices from the pan. Cook, turning the pieces fairly gently, for 3–4 minutes, until the fish is just firm and almost cooked. Push the fish to one side and add the spinach, then cook, stirring it carefully until it has wilted.

Replace the onion and bean mixture and stir all the ingredients together quite gently, allowing the beans and onions to reheat. Taste for seasoning and add more salt and pepper, if necessary. Sprinkle with the spring onions and lemon rind and serve at once.

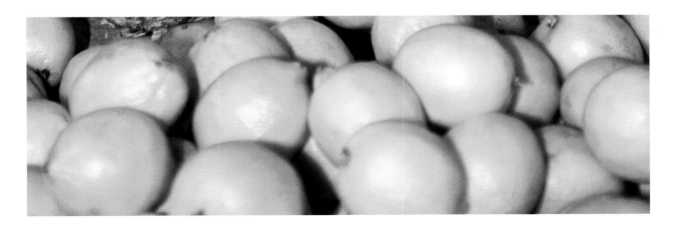

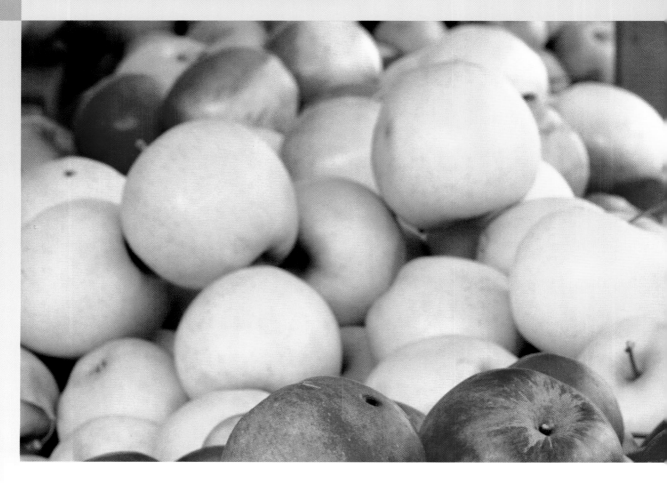

Smoked Mackerel, Apple and Celery Salad with Horseradish and Honey Dressing

On an essential nutritional level, smoked mackerel brings valuable omega-3 fatty acids to the diet but it is also rich in the feel-good factor. It is incredibly easy to prepare – there is no need for cooking or lots of complicated seasoning, just use a fork to flake the succulent flesh off the skin. The flavour bursts through fresh, crisp salad ingredients – such as apple and celery – that complement its natural richness. A punchy horseradish dressing gives this salad an additional kick, and it is traditionally thought to act as a stimulant when eaten, aiding digestion and helping to boost a sluggish system.

Serves 2

4 tablespoons horseradish sauce
2 teaspoons clear honey
150 ml/¼ pint/½ cup Greek-style yogurt or crème fraîche
freshly grated nutmeg
salt and pepper
handful of fresh dill sprigs
4 celery sticks (stalks)
2 crisp, sweet-sour eating apples
wedge of white cabbage
4 spring onions (scallions)
2 smoked mackerel fillets

In a large bowl, mix the horseradish sauce with the honey, then stir in the yogurt or crème fraîche. Season with nutmeg and a little salt and pepper.

Discard any really tough stalks from the dill, then slice the bunch of sprigs and add them to the horseradish dressing. Thinly slice the celery sticks and add them to the bowl. Cut the apples into quarters, remove the cores and slice the quarters across into small pieces. Add the apples to the dressing as they are prepared and turn them in it to prevent them from discolouring.

Finely slice the cabbage so that the wedge separates into shreds. Thinly slice the spring onions. Add both to the bowl and mix well. Finally, pick over the mackerel fillets for any bones and flake the flesh off the skin in chunks. Lightly mix this into the salad and taste for seasoning before serving.

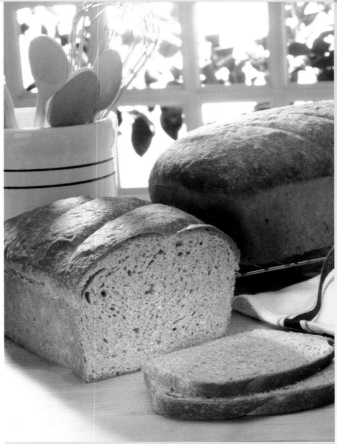

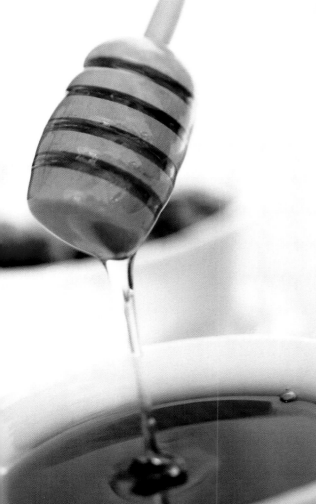

Serving Suggestions

The salad is delicious plain, with lots of warm, crusty wholemeal bread or pitta bread but it can also be offered in a variety of ways.

- Use as a filling for rolls, baguettes or wraps, especially for packed lunches.

- Toss with cold cooked pasta to make a substantial main meal salad.

- Use to fill baked potatoes.

- Brush split ciabatta with a little olive oil and bake until crisp. Top with the salad and serve at once.

- Serve the salad on slices of pan-fried polenta.

Chicken Stir-fry with Broccoli and Beans

Light, swift cooking methods complement a diet rich in vegetables and fruit to contribute to the feeling of vitality. The very process of preparing and cooking this type of dish creates a wonderful sense of wellbeing. The food preparation is relaxing and aromatic, and stir-frying is lively. Using chopsticks or a fork and serving the food from large bowls complements the informal style of dish. Serve with wholegrain rice, couscous or noodles.

Serves 2

2 tablespoons sunflower oil
2 small boneless chicken breasts, cut into fine strips
1 garlic clove, thinly sliced
coarsely grated rind of 1 lime
1 bunch of spring onions (scallions), coarsely chopped
1 red (bell) pepper, seeded and cut into short strips
2 celery sticks (stalks), thinly sliced
100 g/4 oz fine green beans
175 g/6 oz broccoli, cut into small florets
1 tablespoon wholegrain mustard
salt and freshly ground black pepper
100 g/4 oz rocket

Heat the sunflower oil in a wok or large pan. Add the chicken, garlic and lime, and stir-fry until the strips are browned and cooked through, then use a draining spoon to remove them from the pan.

Add the spring onions, pepper, celery, green beans and broccoli to the pan and stir-fry this vegetable mixture for 3–4 minutes, until the vegetables are lightly cooked. Replace the chicken and stir in the mustard with seasoning to taste. Stir-fry for a further 1–2 minutes, until the chicken is reheated.

Finally, sprinkle the rocket into the pan and remove it from the heat. Stir the rocket into the chicken and vegetables and divide it among two bowls.

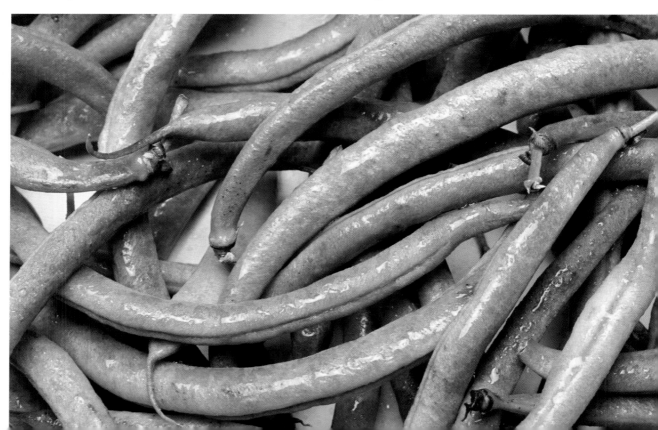

Baked Sweet Potatoes with Cinnamon Stir-fried Chicken

Red-fleshed, carbohydrate-packed sweet potatoes are full of beta carotene in addition to the vitamin C and potassium they provide. With a topping of chicken cooked with warm cinnamon, believed to aid digestion and good circulation, and wonderfully aromatic cumin, a stimulant and diuretic, the result is a meal guaranteed to make you feel full of life. From the colourful appearance and exciting flavours to the nutrients piled on the plate, this dish makes light of the serious business of healthy cooking and great eating.

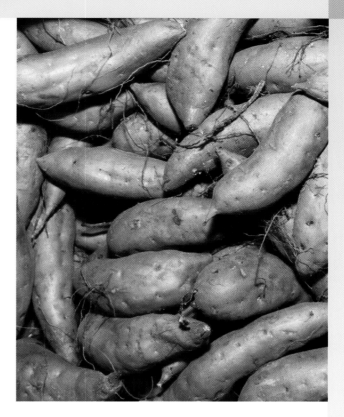

Serves 2

2 small sweet potatoes
2 tablespoons olive oil, plus a little extra for brushing
1 large boneless chicken breast, skinned and cut into thin strips
2 teaspoons ground cinnamon
salt and pepper
1 leek, sliced
1 onion, halved and thinly sliced
1 tablespoon cumin seeds
wedge of white cabbage, shredded
2 carrots, coarsely grated or shredded
grated rind and juice of 1 orange

Preheat the oven to 200°C/400°F/Gas 6. Prick the sweet potatoes, brush them with a little oil and place on a shallow ovenproof dish or tin. Bake the potatoes for 1–1¼ hours, turning once or twice and brushing with a little more oil, if necessary, until they are tender.

Mix the chicken with the cinnamon in a small bowl and set aside to marinate. Begin cooking the chicken mixture 10–15 minutes before the potatoes are ready – timing is not crucial as the potatoes can be left in the oven, with the temperature reduced, without coming to any harm for 10–15 minutes. Heat the oil in a large frying pan (skillet) or wok. Add the chicken with seasoning to taste and stir-fry until the strips are browned. Use a draining spoon to transfer them to a clean plate.

Add the leek, onion and cumin seeds to the oil remaining in the pan, and stir-fry over fairly high heat for 2–3 minutes, until the vegetables are softened. Add the cabbage and carrots and continue to stir-fry briefly until they are hot and well coated in the cooking juices.

Replace the chicken and cook over high heat for a few minutes, stirring, until reheated. Add the orange rind and juice with seasoning to taste. Place the roasted sweet potatoes on plates, split them open and make a few cuts into the tender flesh so that it absorbs the juices from the chicken mixture. Pile the chicken and vegetable mixture on top and serve at once.

Toasted Muffins with Chicken Liver, Bacon and Mushrooms

This flavour-packed light meal is just right for a lunchtime energy boost before a busy afternoon. It is also full of essential nutrients for long-term vitality, particularly iron, A and B-group vitamins and zinc from the liver. Flash-fried green peppers, zingy rocket and shreds of lemon are rejuvenating with the traditional liver and bacon, and they also contribute vitamin C to help the body maximize the goodness in the other ingredients.

Serves 2

2 tablespoons olive oil
2 red (bell) peppers, seeded and sliced
4 spring onions (scallions), cut into short lengths
1 onion, chopped
2 garlic cloves, chopped
2 rindless bacon rashers (slices), diced or cut into strips
½ teaspoon ground mace
4 large sage leaves, thinly shredded
225 g/8 oz/1 cup chicken livers, roughly chopped
salt and pepper
2 wholemeal muffins
150 g/5 oz rocket
coarsely grated rind of 1 lemon, plus lemon wedges to serve
4 tablespoons chopped parsley

Preheat the grill (broiler). Heat the olive oil in a frying pan (skillet). Add the peppers and toss them over high heat for a few seconds, until they are slightly softened and lightly browned in places. Add the spring onions, toss well and then use a slotted spoon to transfer the mixture to a bowl.

Add the onion, garlic and bacon to the oil remaining in the pan and cook, stirring often, until the onion is softened and the bacon cooked and lightly browned. Reduce the heat before adding the mace, sage and chicken livers with a little seasoning. Cook, stirring often, for 3–4 minutes, until livers are firm.

Meanwhile, split and toast the muffins while cooking the livers. Divide the rocket among two plates. Add the lemon rind to the pepper mixture and toss lightly, then spoon this on top of the rocket. Season the salad with freshly ground black pepper and add a lemon wedge to each plate.

Arrange the toasted muffins on the plates. Stir the parsley into the chicken liver mixture and pile it on the muffins. Serve immediately.

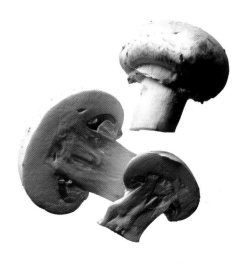

Serving the Chicken Liver Savoury

The chicken liver mixture is versatile and delicious in all sorts of guises. Try some of the following for super-healthy meals or snacks.

- Pile the mixture in large fluffy, crisp-skinned baked potatoes.

- Toss the chicken livers and pepper salad with freshly cooked pasta.

- Top cooked rice or couscous with the salad, then add the chicken liver mixture.

- For a delicious packed lunch, allow the chicken liver mixture to cool, then dress it with a little lemon juice. Fill a split baguette with the pepper salad and the chicken liver mixture. Wrap in cling film (saran wrap).

- Use the chicken liver mixture as a filling for an omelette.

- Roll up the chicken liver mixture in warm wheat tortilla wraps and serve with the salad.

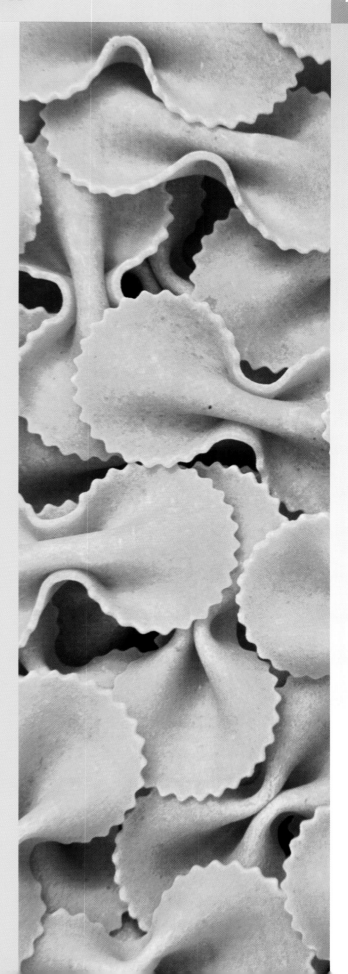

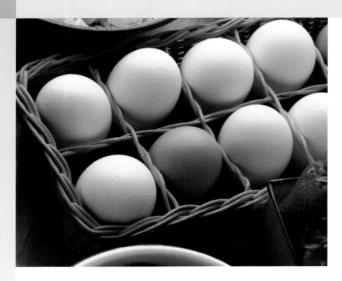

Tomato and Tarragon Risotto with Poached Eggs in Chilli and Caper Dressing

Sweet, gentle and delicious tomato risotto explodes into irresistible life when topped with soft poached eggs coated with an exhilarating dressing of tarragon and capers. Serve a crisp salad, with plenty of finely sliced peppers, to bring the smooth textures of this taste-bud-tingling dish to life. Add some crusty wholegrain bread for additional complex carbohydrate as a source of long-term energy.

Serves 4

575 g/1¼lb tomatoes, peeled and halved
6 tablespoons olive oil
1 large onion, finely chopped
1 garlic clove, crushed
225 g/8oz/1¼ cup risotto rice
salt and pepper
250 ml/8fl oz/1 cup white wine
(preferably medium dry but dry will do)
600 ml/1 pint/2½ cups hot chicken or vegetable stock
1 teaspoon sugar
4 tablespoons chopped tarragon
1 mild green chilli, seeded and thinly sliced
2 tablespoons coarsely chopped capers
2 tablespoons snipped chives
4–8 eggs

Scoop the middles out of the tomatoes and sieve the pulp, discarding the seeds. Finely dice the tomato shells and set them aside separately from the pulp.

Heat 2 tablespoons of the oil in a large saucepan. Add the onion and garlic, and cook, stirring occasionally, until the onion has softened slightly. Stir in the rice to coat the grains in oil. Add the tomato pulp, salt and pepper and wine, and bring to the boil. Reduce the heat and simmer, uncovered, until the liquid is absorbed.

Add about half the stock, bring to simmering point and stir. Simmer until the stock has all been absorbed, then add the remaining stock and continue simmering until it too has been absorbed. Stir in the diced tomatoes, sugar and tarragon, cover and set the pan aside off the heat.

Pour the remaining oil into a small saucepan and add the chilli. Cook over gentle heat for 1 minute, then add the capers and chives with a little seasoning. Cover the pan and set it aside off the heat. The heat of the pan should be sufficient to keep the dressing warm while the eggs are cooking.

Poach the eggs until the whites are just set or cooked to taste. Alternatively, soft-boil the eggs for 4–5 minutes and shell them carefully – the whites should be firm and the yolks lightly set after 5 minutes. Divide the risotto between four warm serving bowls. Top the risotto with the eggs and spoon the dressing over. Serve at once.

Fresh Pasta with Shredded Herb Omelette, Courgettes and Cherry Tomatoes

This is simple, carbohydrate-rich supper dish is full of lively flavours and ingredients that help to promote vitality.

Serves 2

450 g/1 lb cherry tomatoes, halved
4 tablespoons olive oil
4 garlic cloves, sliced
4 small courgettes (zucchini), thinly sliced
10 black olives, pitted and thinly sliced
225 g/8 oz fresh pasta shapes
salt and pepper
4 eggs
4 spring onions (scallions), finely chopped
2 tablespoons chopped coriander (cilantro)
1 tablespoon chopped tarragon
2 tablespoons chopped thyme
4 tablespoons chopped parsley

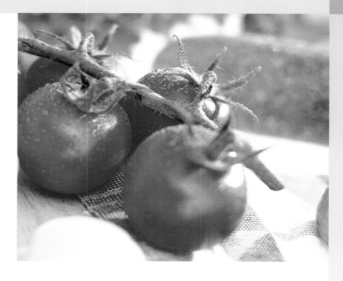

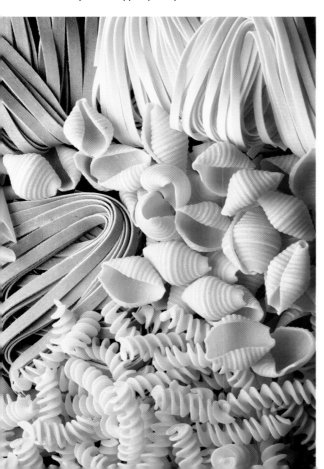

Place the tomatoes in a large bowl. Gently heat 3 tablespoons of the oil in a large frying pan (skillet) or saucepan and add the garlic. Allow the garlic to sizzle gently for a few minutes, then add the courgettes and toss well over high heat for about 1 minute, until the courgettes are lightly cooked. Add the courgettes, oil and garlic to the tomatoes with the olives.

Bring a large saucepan of salted water to the boil for cooking the pasta. Add the pasta and bring back to the boil, then cook according to the packet instructions for about 3–5 minutes, depending on the type and size of pasta.

Meanwhile, beat the eggs with seasoning. Then add the spring onions, coriander, tarragon, thyme and parsley. Heat the remaining oil in a large frying pan and pour in the egg mixture. Cook the eggs until set around the edge, then lift the omelette and allow uncooked egg to run underneath. As soon as the omelette is set, slide it out on to a plate and shred it into fine strips.

Drain the pasta and add it to the courgette and tomato mixture. Add the shredded omelette and toss lightly. Serve at once.

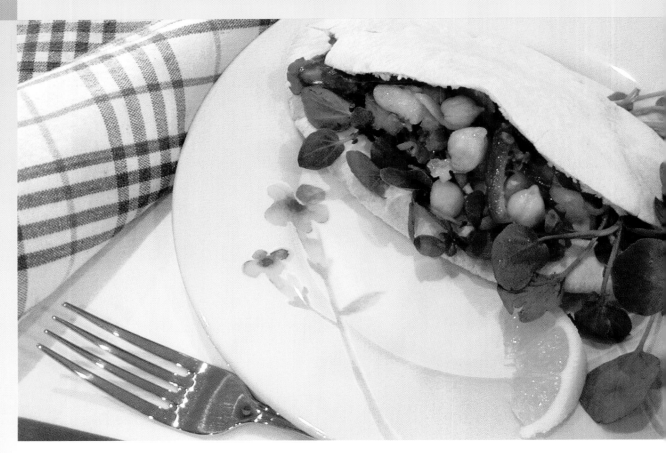

Watercress and Chickpea Salad in Pitta

This makes an excellent and substantial snack for lunch or supper, providing plenty of vitamins and minerals along with protein and complex carbohydrate. The combination of lively flavours and bulky watercress with slightly astringent green pepper is invigorating – just the food to wake up the taste buds and bring a zing to life. Follow on with a piece of fruit or fruit salad and yogurt, or have a fresh fruit juice or smoothie with the stuffed pitta.

Serves 4

400 g/14 oz can chickpeas, drained
1 tablespoon olive oil
1 garlic clove, chopped
1 green (bell) pepper, seeded and finely diced
grated rind of 1 lemon and juice of ½ lemon
2 spring onions (scallions), chopped

50 g/2 oz/¼ cup medjool or fresh dates, pitted and sliced
8 pitta bread
100 g/4 oz watercress sprigs

Place the chickpeas in a bowl and coarsely crush about a third of them with a fork. Add the olive oil, garlic, pepper, lemon rind and juice, spring onions and dates. Mix the ingredients thoroughly, encouraging the crushed chickpeas to absorb the oil and lemon juice so that the salad clings together.

Warm the pitta bread under a hot grill (broiler) for about 30 seconds on each side until they are slightly puffed. Then slit them and pack with the watercress and the salad. Serve at once or wrap each filled bread in cling film (saran wrap) if they are being prepared for a packed lunch.

Strawberry, Lime and Pecan Cream Layer

This simple, fruit and nut mixture is just as good for breakfast as it is for dessert. Vary and mix the fruit according to what is available – strawberries are thought of as a cleansing and enlivening fruit, providing a tonic. With zesty lime, honey and nuts this makes a satisfying and energy-boosting snack.

Serves 4

450 g/1 lb/2 cups low-fat fromage frais
grated rind and juice of 1 lime
4 teaspoons clear honey, or to taste
100 g/4 oz/1 cup oat flakes
100 g/4 oz/½ cup pecan nuts, coarsely chopped
450 g/1 lb/2½ cups strawberries, hulled and halved

Mix the fromage frais with the lime rind and juice, and half the honey. Heat a large heavy frying pan (skillet) and add the oat flakes. Dry roast them over medium heat, stirring continuously, until they smell toasted and are lightly browned in places. Transfer to a bowl and add the pecan nuts and remaining honey.

Reserve 8 strawberry halves for decoration. Layer the remaining strawberries, fromage frais, and oat and pecan mixture in four large glasses or dishes. Top with the reserved strawberries and serve.

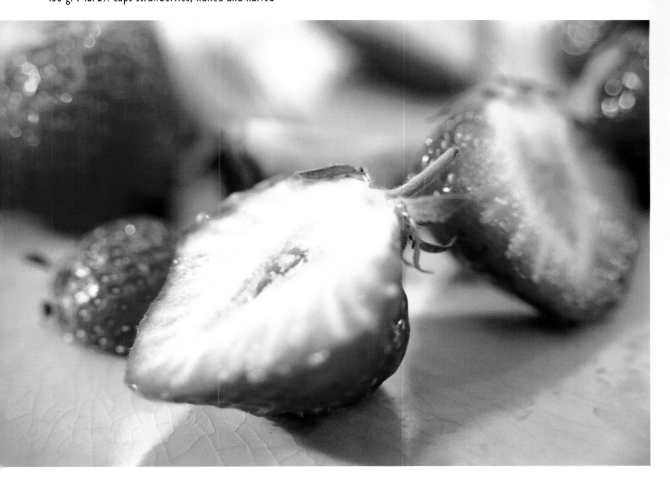

Ginger-Laced Banana and Blueberry Yogurt

Mild, delicious and satisfying are the words to describe this luscious, sweet mixture which makes a brilliantly nutritious breakfast or a great dessert after a light main course. It is also the perfect pick-me-up for those moments when the energy gap seems to fill the afternoon. Chopped candied ginger is readily available and a good alternative to the more expensive stem ginger preserved in syrup. It sweetens and enlivens this fruit mixture, bringing that zesty twist towards vigour and vitality.

Serves 2

3 tablespoons chopped candied ginger
300 ml/½ pint/1 cup plain yogurt
100 g/4 oz/⅔ cup blueberries
2 bananas
4 tablespoons chopped hazelnuts

Mix the ginger into the yogurt until evenly distributed, then taste the yogurt for sweetness and add a little extra ginger, if liked. Mix in the blueberries. Slice the bananas, add them to the yogurt mixture. Stir, then divide mixture between two bowls. Sprinkle with the hazelnuts and serve at once.

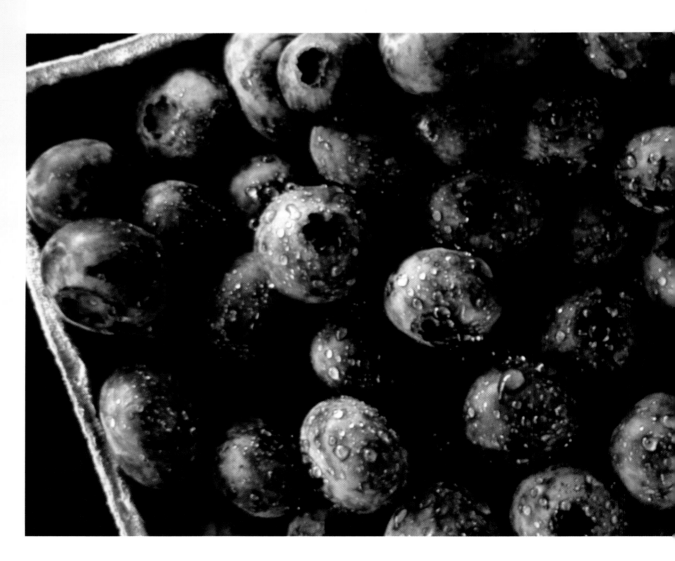

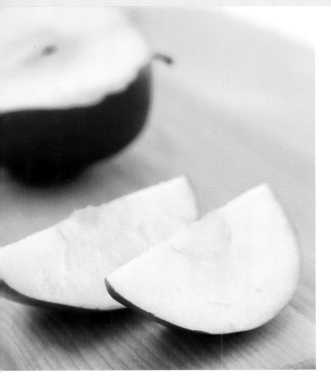

Three-Fruit, Sunflower and Pine Nut Muesli

No collection of ideas on foods for vitality would be complete without muesli. The commercial cereals full of sugar, lots of dried fruit, nuts and dried milk powder can be dismally distant from anything that promotes a wide-awake feeling first thing in the morning. This lively, fresh fruit and grain mixture with toasted sunflower seeds and pine nuts is light and palate cleansing. At the same time, it is sufficiently sustaining to provide a source of energy that will see you through the very worst of mornings.

Serves 2

4 tablespoons sunflower seeds

4 tablespoons pine nuts

4 tablespoons rye flakes

4 tablespoons barley flakes

4 tablespoons bran

4 tablespoons oat flakes

4 ready-to-eat dried peaches, sliced, snipped or chopped into pieces

2 dessert apples, cored and diced

100 g/4 oz/1 cup seedless green grapes

apple juice, milk or yogurt to serve

Heat a heavy frying pan (skillet) and dry roast the sunflower seeds over low to medium heat, stirring continuously, until lightly browned. Transfer to a bowl, then roast the pine nuts, rye flakes and barley flakes separately. Add each batch to the bowl immediately it is cooked. Wipe the pan out with kitchen paper after roasting the rye flakes, before adding the barley, as any cooked, floury residue will begin to burn and turn bitter by the time the next batch of flakes is ready.

Stir in the bran and oat flakes. Then add the peaches, diced apple and grapes. The grapes can be left whole – in which case they bring exciting bursts of sweet-sour juiciness to the mixture when eaten – or halved for an even distribution of their flavour. Make sure all the ingredients are thoroughly combined, then pile the mueseli into large, deep bowls. Serve with unsweetened apple juice, milk or yogurt.

Roasted Seeded Muesli

This is my favourite seed and grain mix and one that I put to all sorts of uses: I sprinkle it on fruit salad, as here, for breakfast or a quick snack; add it to bread; cook it with a little bacon or chorizo sausage to make a delicious salad or soup garnish; or use it as a topping for gratins or sweet fruit bakes. The seeds are bursting with minerals, protein and omega-3 fatty acids. The grains provide plenty of complex carbohydrate for slow-release energy at the start of the day.

Serves 2

1 teaspoon fennel seeds
1 teaspoon linseeds
2 tablespoons sesame seeds
2 tablespoons sunflower seeds
2 tablespoons pumpkin seeds
4 tablespoons barley flakes
4 tablespoons rye flakes
4 tablespoons oatflakes
4 tablespoons rolled oats or millet
1 apple, cored and diced
2 kiwi fruit, peeled and diced or 100 g/4 oz/1 cup seedless grapes
1 orange, peeled, seeded and roughly chopped
100 g/4 oz/⅔ cup blueberries
300 ml/½ pint/1 cup plain yogurt
a little honey or maple syrup (optional)

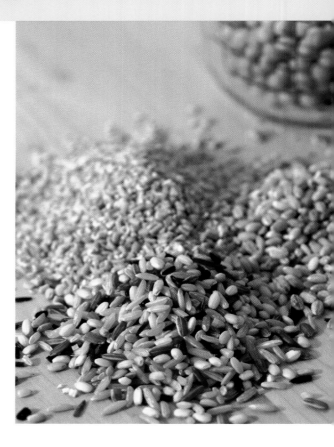

In a heavy, dry frying pan (skillet), roast the fennel and linseeds together over medium heat until the fennel smells aromatic and they begin to pop. Immediately tip them out of the pan into a bowl. Roast the sesame seeds next, followed by the sunflower and then the pumpkin seeds. Take care to keep the heat moderate to low so as not to burn the seeds and tip them out of the pan at once, or they will continue to cook in the residual heat.

Roast the barley, rye and oat flakes separately or together, depending on the size of pan, as if it is too full it will be difficult to avoid overcooking the grains. Mix the seeds and grains, then leave to cool.

Toss the prepared fruit together and add the seeds and grains. Divide the mixture between two bowls and top with yogurt. Drizzle with a little honey or maple syrup, if liked and serve at once.

Caraway, Cashew and Apricot Flapjacks

Flapjacks are full of complex carbohydrate from the oats, as well as sugar for a short-term energy boost. This recipe makes the most of the positive contribution from dried apricots, buttery cashew nuts and enlivening caraway seeds. One of these makes an excellent treat for breakfast at weekends, getting the day off to a good start. Have a healthy fresh fruit drink or fruit salad to complete the meal.

Makes 16

100 g/4 oz/½ cup butter
6 tablespoons clear honey
grated rind and juice of 1 orange
2 tablespoons caraway seeds
150 g/5 oz/⅔ cup ready-to-eat dried apricots, chopped
100 g/4 oz/½ cup unsalted plain cashew nuts, roughly chopped
225 g/8 oz/1 cup rolled oats
4 tablespoons bran

Preheat the oven to 190°C/375°F/Gas 5 and grease a 20 cm/8 in square tin. Mix the butter and honey with the orange rind and juice, caraway seeds and apricots in a large saucepan. Stir over medium heat until the butter has melted.

Remove the pan from the heat and mix in the cashew nuts, oats and bran. Stir until the ingredients are thoroughly combined and all the oats and bran are moistened. Turn the mixture into the prepared tin and press it down evenly and firmly with the back of a metal spoon.

Bake the flapjacks for about 20 minutes, or until the mixture is golden brown on top and darker around the edges. Leave the mixture to cool for 10 minutes, then cut it into sixteen flapjacks. Leave the flapjacks to cool and set before using a flexible plastic spatula to remove them from the tin. Store in an airtight container.

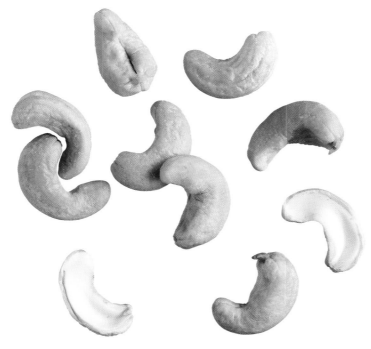

Food is familiar as a restorative during times of physical stress, weakness or illness. In this traditional sense, light, nutritious foods provide the body with the nourishment it needs to counteract the demands placed on it or to rebuild and repair damage. The innate response to eating in this sense is also closely linked to its ability to comfort and reassure, especially when the appetite is lost and eating may be physically difficult as, for example, when suffering from a bad cold or sore throat.

Although we do not think about it, eating is an ongoing process of restoring the body – replacing used nutrients, replenishing energy supplies, and encouraging growth and repair. Previous generations that experienced food shortages, limited choice and real hardship – to the extent of not being able to afford enough food to live on – paid real attention to the ingredients of every meal, but today we tend to take our food for granted.

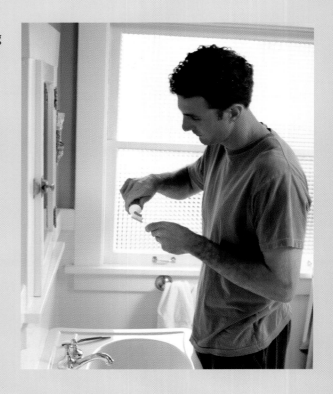

Meals are often barely noticed or acknowledged as anything other than another essential act in the day, on a par with washing the face or cleaning the teeth. Indeed, the amount of attention paid to appearance suggests that eating comes far lower down the scale of importance than face care. Beyond the idea of snacking or grazing, or grabbing the nearest edible convenience product between social or work windows in the day, food has joined the ranks of other fashion accessories. This worst-case scenario consists of dismissing food as the simplest and least offensive item to fulfil a physical need on one hand and using it as a status symbol or fashion statement on the other.

In reality, food, the way in which it is cooked, and our attitude to meals can all restore or provide a boost in far more than the physical sense. As a whole, this type of nourishment feeds the mind and spirit as well as the body.

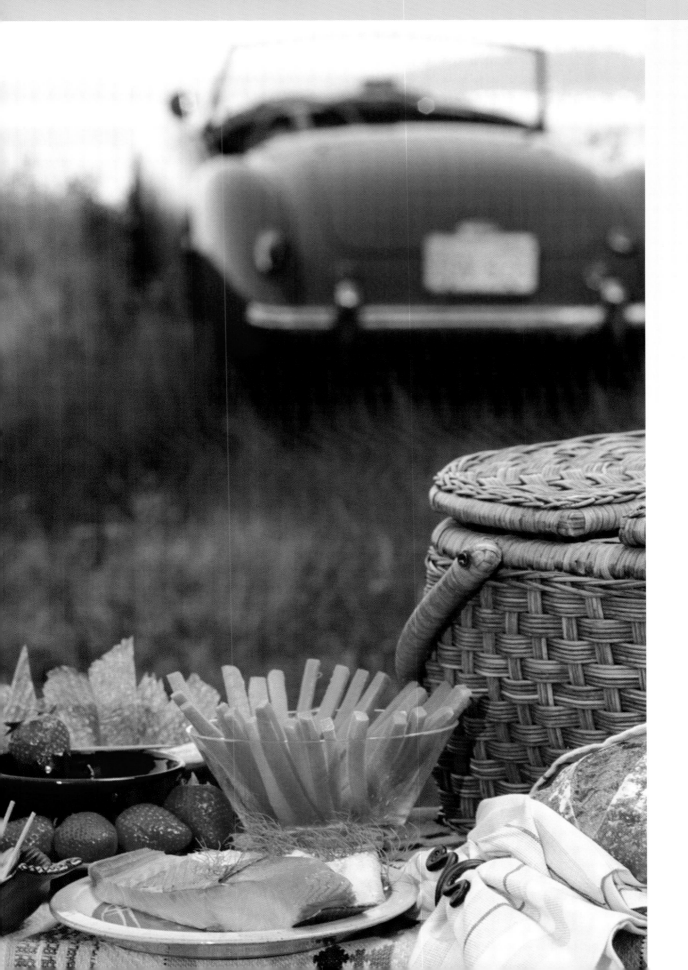

Herbed Chicken and Vegetable Broth

This simple soup is full of herbs that have long been valued as stimulants, tonics and aids to digestion – parsley, sage, thyme and tarragon all have strong associations as medicinal herbs. This is a light broth that is easy to eat while providing protein, vitamins and minerals from the chicken and vegetables. There are many other ways of making chicken soups, using portions on the bone or the leftovers from a roast, but the emphasis here is on simple, modern cooking. Making this soup is effortless and it will boost the spirit and restore enthusiasm for caring and nurturing a sense of wellbeing.

Serves 4

2 tablespoons sunflower oil
350 g/12 oz skinless, boneless chicken meat (such as diced, stir-fry strips or boneless breast fillet), diced if necessary
4 bay leaves
1 large onion, halved and thinly sliced
1 large leek, halved lengthwise and thinly sliced
4 celery sticks (stalks), halved lengthwise and thinly sliced
2 large carrots, quartered lengthwise and thinly sliced
4 large sage sprigs, stalks discarded and leaves finely shredded
4 large tarragon sprigs, stalks discarded and leaves finely shredded
leaves from 4 large thyme sprigs
1.12 litres/2 pints/5 cups water
1 green (bell) pepper, seeded and diced
salt and pepper
1 large broccoli spear, tender stalk diced and head broken into small florets
good handful of tender parsley sprigs, chopped

Heat the oil in a large saucepan. Add the chicken and stir until the pieces are separated and browned. Add the bay leaves, onion, leek, celery, carrots, sage, tarragon and thyme leaves. Stir well, cover the pan and cook over low to medium heat for 15 minutes, until the vegetables are softened slightly but not browned.

Pour in the water and add the green pepper with seasoning to taste, then bring to the boil. Reduce the heat, cover the pan and simmer gently for 30 minutes. Taste the soup and add more seasoning, if necessary. Stir in the broccoli, bring back to the boil and reduce the heat again. Cover and simmer for 5 minutes. Add the parsley and taste for seasoning, then serve the soup piping hot.

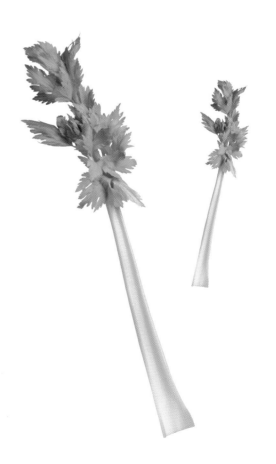

Creamy Roasted Garlic, Leek and Onion Soup

Onions, leeks and garlic belong to the allium family of vegetables that has an ancient reputation for restorative and healing qualities. In folk medicine, onions are thought of as a vegetable for curing and preventing illness, and modern research into the role of vegetables in the diet supports the value of onions and their relatives. French onion soup is a traditionally restorative dish but this contemporary soup is quite different. The sweet and soothing flavours of roasted garlic and onions are balanced by refreshing leeks and the whole potful is thickened with oatmeal for useful complex carbohydrate. The aroma, texture and flavour of the soup all contribute to the pleasure it brings – make it on a cold day and savour the warmth it imparts.

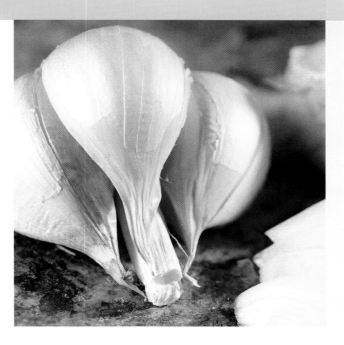

Serves 4

2 large unpeeled onions

1 whole bulb of garlic

3 tablespoons olive oil

4 bay leaves

3 leeks, sliced

salt and pepper

1.12 litres/2 pints/5 cups chicken stock

6 tablespoons fine oatmeal

150 ml/¼ pint/⅔ cup crème fraîche

grated rind of 1 lemon

large handful of parsley sprigs, chopped

Preheat the oven to 200°C/400°F/Gas 6. Brush the unpeeled onions and bulb of garlic with a little of the oil and place in a small dish. Roast for 30 minutes. Remove the garlic and replace the onions in the oven for a further 10–15 minutes, or until they are tender.

Pour the remaining olive oil into a large saucepan. Add the bay leaves and heat gently until the leaves begin to sizzle. Add the leeks and seasoning, stir well, cover and cook for about 15 minutes, until the leeks are greatly reduced and tender.

Meanwhile, remove the outer peel from the head of garlic, separate the cloves and squeeze their flesh into the pan with the leeks. Use a serrated knife to slit the onions open and scoop the soft flesh into the pan with the leeks. Stir well. Pour in the stock and bring to the boil. Reduce the heat, cover the pan and simmer for 20 minutes.

Sprinkle the oatmeal into the soup, stirring all the time, then bring to the boil, stirring. Reduce the heat and cover the pan again, then simmer for a further 5 minutes. Cool the soup slightly and pick out the bay leaves before puréeing in a blender. Return the soup to the pan and stir in the cream. Taste for seasoning and reheat gently without boiling.

Ladle the soup into large bowls. Mix the lemon rind and parsley and sprinkle generous amounts over the soup. Serve at once.

Pan-fried Plaice with Fennel Seeds and Lemon

This is supremely simple and appetite arousing – just the recipe for a light meal to boost the system. Serve with new potatoes and stir-fried carrots with Chinese greens (pak choi) to make a well-balanced, light and bright meal. Fennel is an aid to digestion, an appetite stimulant and general tonic to improve a sluggish system (the seeds are used to make an infusion or tea that can be drunk to relieve wind and act as a general tonic).

Serves 2

2 teaspoons fennel seeds
2 tablespoons olive oil
2 large plaice fillets
salt and pepper
coarsely grated rind and juice of ½ lemon
2 tablespoons chopped fennel (optional)

Gently heat the fennel seeds in a large frying pan (skillet) with the oil, keeping the heat low so that the oil barely moves around the seeds.

Season the plaice fillets. Slightly increase the heat under the pan so that the seeds are just sizzling, then add the plaice fillets, skin uppermost. Cook until lightly browned, then use a large slice to turn the fillets over, picking up as many of the fennel seeds as possible. Increase the heat and cook the fish on the second side until the skin is browned and crisped.

Transfer the plaice to warmed plates. Add the lemon rind and juice to the pan and bring to the boil, stirring. Boil briefly, stirring, until the juice is reduced, then pour it over the fish and sprinkle with the fennel, if using. Serve immediately.

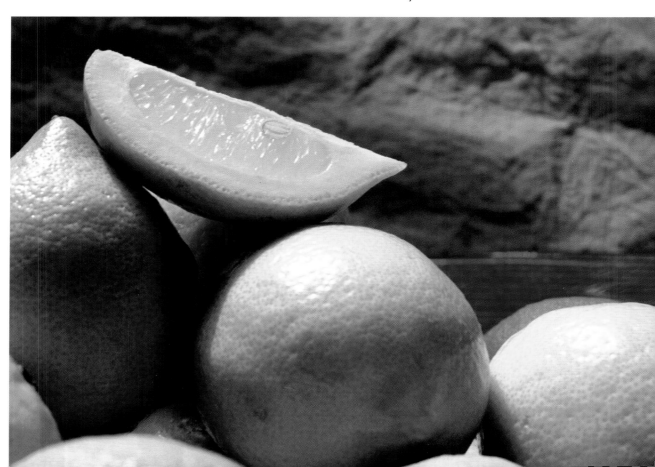

Simply Succulent Venison with Apple and Red Cabbage

This is an excellent feel-good dish of marinated lean venison which is deliciously special with a fruity combination of apple, raisins and red cabbage. For a physical boost, the lean venison provides iron and B vitamins, while the apples and cabbage contribute vitamin C to help the body make the most of the iron content of the meat. Aromatic juniper and caraway contribute their traditional properties as stimulants with characteristic uplifting and appetizing aromas and warmth.

Serves 4

1 tablespoon juniper berries, crushed

1 tablespoon caraway seeds

1 garlic clove, thinly sliced

4 bay leaves

2 tablespoons raisins

300 ml/½ pint/1¼ cups unsweetened apple juice

4 venison escalopes, about 175 g/6 oz each

salt and pepper

2 tablespoons sunflower oil

1 small onion, finely chopped

350 g/12 oz red cabbage, finely shredded

4 dessert apples, peeled, cored and diced

2 tablespoons cider vinegar

2 tablespoons crab apple or redcurrant jelly

apple wedges to garnish (optional)

Heat the juniper berries, caraway seeds, garlic, bay leaves, raisins and apple juice in a small saucepan until the juice boils. Simmer for 2 minutes, then set aside to cool completely.

Place the venison escalopes in a small deep dish and pour in the cold spice and apple juice mixture. Turn the escalopes in the juices so that they are evenly coated. Cover and leave to marinate for anything from a couple of hours to a day.

Drain the escalopes well, scraping off all the spice residue back into the marinade. Pat the meat dry on kitchen paper, then season the escalopes. Warm the grill (broiler) compartment and a dish ready to keep the cooked meat hot. Heat half the oil in a large, deep, preferably non-stick, heavy frying pan (skillet). Cook the venison escalopes quickly over high heat for about 3 minutes on each side, until well browned. Transfer to the warm plate, cover with foil and keep hot.

Add the remaining oil to the pan and fry the onion over high heat until beginning to brown in places. Add the cabbage and apple and cook, stirring, until slightly tender – do not allow the cabbage to become soft. Pour the vinegar over the cabbage and cook for a few seconds, then add the crab apple or redcurrant jelly and pour in the reserved marinade. Cook over high heat, turning and stirring the cabbage, until the liquor is reduced and the cabbage is well glazed.

Transfer the cabbage and apple mixture to serving plates, reserving the bay leaves for garnish. Cut the venison escalopes into wide strips and arrange them on top of the cabbage. Pour over any juices that may have seeped from the venison and garnish with the reserved bay leaves and apples (if using). Serve immediately.

Hot Duck Fillets with Orange and Ginger on Watercress and Kiwi Salad

Duck breast fillets are readily available, quick to prepare and cook and they provide a good source of iron, potassium, zinc and the B vitamins. Zesty orange and ginger go especially well with the rich, dry flavour of the meat, as does the kiwi fruit. Kiwi fruit is rich in vitamin C and its slightly tangy grape-like flavour is delicious with savoury ingredients. Serve this hot-cold salad with plenty of crusty wholemeal bread, brown rice or baked potatoes for complex carbohydrate to provide plenty of energy. Allow the wonderful mix of flavours and textures, and the simple contemporary style of the food to restore and boost your enthusiasm for life.

Serves 2

2 skinless boneless duck breasts
grated rind and juice of 1 orange
15 g/½ oz fresh root ginger, peeled and finely chopped
1 tablespoon honey
1 tablespoon sunflower oil
salt and pepper
150 g/5 oz watercress
handful of flat-leaf parsley leaves
4 spring onions, sliced
2 kiwi fruit, peeled, halved and sliced

Place the duck in a small bowl and add the orange rind and juice, ginger and honey. Turn the duck in the flavouring mixture to coat the pieces evenly, then cover the dish and leave to marinate for 1–2 hours if possible.

Drain the duck, reserving the marinade. Season the duck well on both sides. Heat the oil in a non-stick frying pan (skillet) and add the duck. Cook over high heat for 3–5 minutes on each side, until the duck is browned and cooked through.

Meanwhile, mix the watercress, parsley, spring onions and kiwi fruit and divide this salad among two bowls or plates. Transfer the cooked duck to a plate and pour the reserved marinade into the pan. Bring to the boil and cook, stirring, for a few seconds to remove all the residue from the pan. Remove from the heat.

Slice the duck breasts and arrange them on the salad, then dress with the cooking juices and marinade in the pan. Serve immediately.

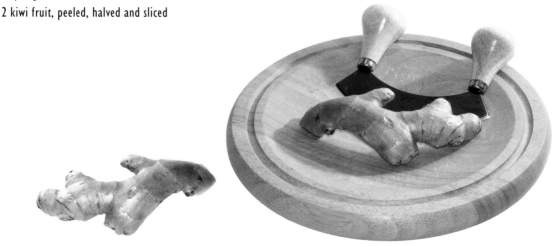

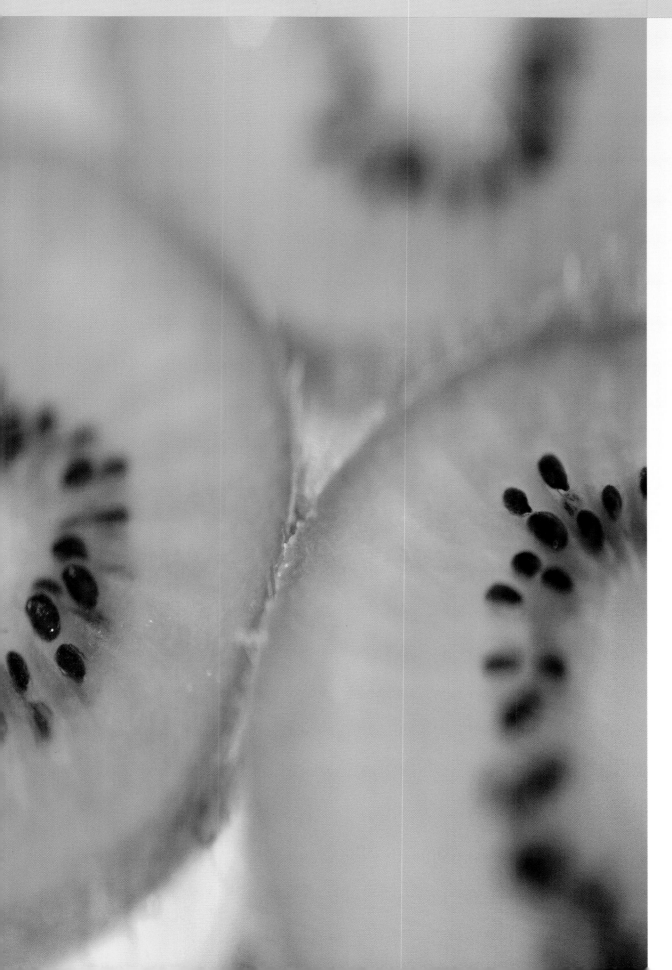

Coriander-spiced Scrambled Eggs with Tomatoes, Watercress and Basil

Scrambled eggs are nutritious and easy to eat. Here they are complemented by stimulating coriander (an aid to digestion) as well as tomatoes, watercress and basil for a folate boost and vitamin C that helps iron absorption. The aesthetics of the dish are especially important – the warm, creamy eggs are balanced by fresh and uplifting tomatoes, watercress and sunny basil. With crunchy wholegrain toast dressed with olive oil instead of butter, the result is a deliciously light and healthy meal or substantial weekend breakfast.

Serves 1

2 slices Granary bread or seeded wholegrain bread
2 tablespoons olive oil
1 tablespoon coriander (cilantro) seeds, crushed
salt and pepper
2 eggs
2 tomatoes, diced
2 large basil sprigs, thinly shredded
large handful of watercress, coarsely chopped

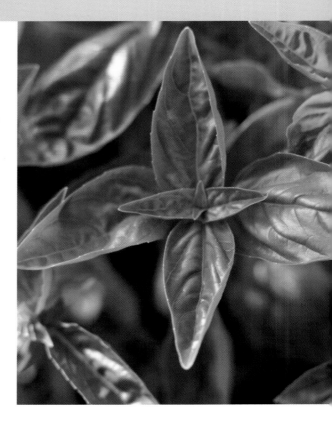

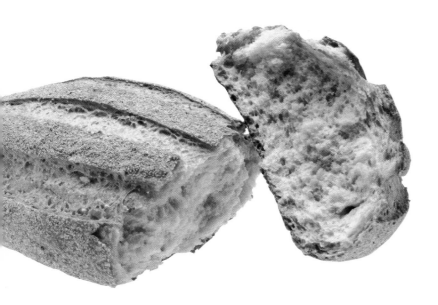

Toast the bread slices on one side, then brush the second sides evenly, using 1 tablespoon of the olive oil. Place the bread, oil sides up, well away from the heat under the grill (broiler) so that they brown very slowly and evenly while you are cooking the eggs. Check the bread frequently as you continue to cook the eggs and reduce the grill heat or turn it off when the slices are golden.

Heat the remaining oil and crushed coriander seeds in a small, heavy saucepan and allow the coriander to sizzle gently for about 30 seconds or until aromatic. Remove from the heat and allow to cool slightly. Season the eggs and whisk until frothy on the surface.

Pour the mixture into the coriander and oil in the pan. Replace the pan over low heat and cook, whisking or stirring continuously, until the eggs are lightly set. Stop whisking and stir in the tomatoes. Cook briefly until the tomatoes are hot and the eggs creamy.

Do not overcook at this stage or the eggs and tomatoes will become watery. Remove from the heat as soon as the eggs are creamy. Add the basil and taste for seasoning.

Place the toasted bread on a warm plate and top with the watercress. Pile the eggs and tomatoes on top and serve immediately.

Microwave cooking

The scrambled eggs and tomatoes are even better cooked in the microwave. Toast the bread as in the main recipe. Roast the coriander seeds in a dry pan until they are aromatic before crushing them, alternatively use ½ teaspoon of ground coriander instead. Beat the eggs with the olive oil, coriander and seasoning in a bowl suitable for microwave cooking. Place the tomatoes in a bowl suitable for microwave cooking and heat them for 30–60 seconds, until they are just hot but not cooked; set aside. Microwave the eggs for intervals of 30 seconds, whisking in between, until they are lightly set. Leave to stand for about 30 seconds, by which time the eggs should be creamy. If necessary, heat the tomatoes again while the eggs are standing. Stir the tomatoes and basil into the eggs. Finish as in the main recipe.

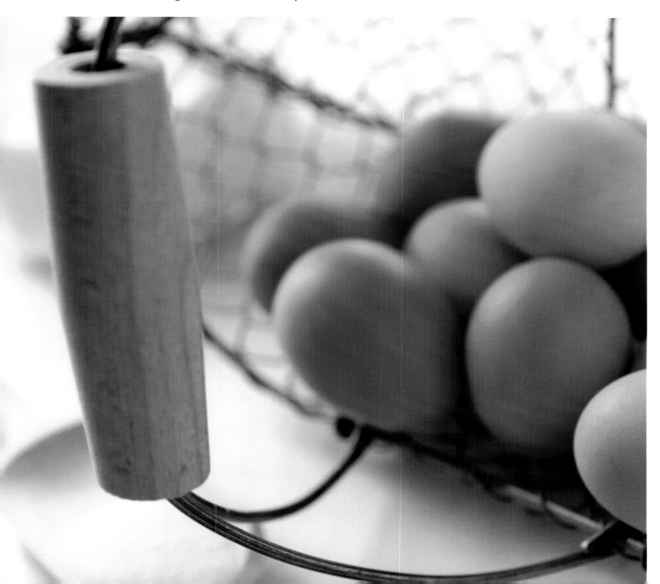

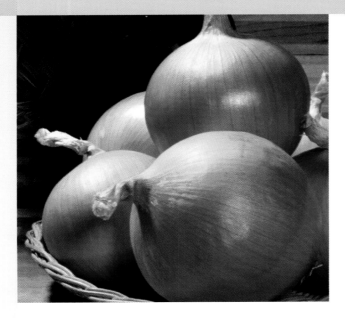

Glazed Onion Tart with Sage-scented Parmesan Pastry

Succulent little onions cooked to deep-golden perfection are delicious in a simple, creamy quiche. The pastry is crisp and savoury with a modest amount of full-flavoured Parmesan and warming, uplifting fresh sage. A combination of wholemeal and plain flour brings complex carbohydrate for a sustained boost to energy. Serve with a salad of baby plum tomatoes or cherry tomatoes tossed with lively chives, heartwarming basil and lots of rocket to make an accompaniment that is rich in vitamin C.

Serves 6

100 g/4 oz/1 cup wholemeal flour
50 g/2 oz/½ cup plain (all-purpose) flour
75 g/3 oz/6 tablespoons butter
50 g/2 oz/⅔ cup freshly grated Parmesan cheese
leaves from 1 large sage sprig, chopped
2 tablespoons sunflower oil
450 g/1 lb pickling onions
salt and pepper
1 teaspoon sugar
3 eggs
300 ml/½ pint/1¼ cups milk
freshly grated nutmeg

Mix the wholemeal and plain flours, then rub in the butter until the mixture resembles fine breadcrumbs. This mixture can be processed in a food processor until fine. Mix in the Parmesan cheese and sage, then add 3 tablespoons of water and bring the mixture together into a short pastry dough. Roll out the pastry and use to line a 23 cm/10 in flan dish (pie tin). Chill in the freezer for 15 minutes or for 30 minutes in the fridge.

Preheat the oven to 200°C/400°F/Gas 6. Prick the base all over, then line the pastry case with greaseproof (waxed) paper and sprinkle with baking beans or dried beans. Bake for 15 minutes, then remove from the oven. Reduce the oven temperature to 180°C/350°F/Gas 4. Remove the paper and beans from the pastry case and place the dish or tin on a baking sheet so that it is easier to lift when filled.

While the pastry case is being chilled and baked blind, prepare the filling. Heat the oil in a large saucepan and add the pickling onions with a little seasoning. Cook over medium heat, stirring occasionally, until the onions are tender and beginning to brown. Sprinkle with the sugar and continue to cook until evenly and lightly browned. Spread the cooked onions out in the pastry case.

Beat the eggs with the milk, seasoning and a little grated nutmeg. Pour this mixture into the quiche around the onions. Bake the quiche for about 40 minutes, until the filling is set and well browned. Serve hot or warm.

Baked Papaya with Spiced Walnut and Angelica Filling

Papaya and walnuts provide an excellent supply of health-giving nutrients, including minerals, vitamin C, beta carotene from the fruit, and B vitamins and antioxidant vitamin E from the nuts. Angelica stems, seeds and leaves are thought to have stimulant and tonic qualities and are an aid to digestion. Appreciating the impact food makes on health contributes to a positive feeling about preparing it, cooking and eating, that in turn encourages a general sense of enthusiasm for a diet to promote wellbeing.

Serves 2

2 papaya, halved, seeded and peeled
grated rind and juice of ½ lime
1 tablespoon sunflower oil
1 teaspoon ground ginger
1 teaspoon ground cinnamon
¼ teaspoon grated nutmeg
1 tablespoon soft (light) brown sugar
4 tablespoons finely chopped candied angelica
4 tablespoons finely chopped walnuts
4 tablespoons fresh wholemeal breadcrumbs
fromage frais or yogurt to serve

Set the oven at 190°C/375°F/Gas 9. Roll up four pieces of foil into thin sausage shapes and use them to support the papaya halves in an ovenproof dish.

Mix the lime rind and juice with the sunflower oil, ginger, cinnamon, nutmeg and brown sugar. Stir in the angelica and walnuts. Mix in the breadcrumbs, turning them with the other ingredients and juices until they are evenly moistened.

Spoon the mixture into the papaya halves, piling it up on them. Bake for about 20 minutes, until the filling is browned. Serve hot or warm, with fromage frais or yogurt.

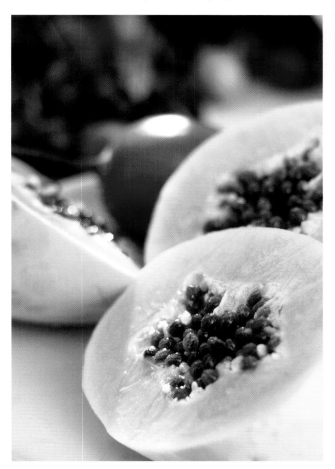

Spiced Light Apple Fool

This light fruit fool is supremely simple and reassuring to make and eat. It is full of the goodness of fruit and stimulating with cloves and cinnamon. Serve it straight as a dessert or with porridge, or topped with a generous sprinkling of Essential Seeds and Grains for breakfast.

Serves 4

1 cinnamon stick
6 cloves
100 ml/4 fl oz/½ cup water
grated rind and juice of 1 lemon
450 g/1 lb full-flavoured cooking apples
75 g/3 oz/⅓ cup soft (light) brown sugar
450 g/1 lb/2 cups low-fat fromage frais

Place the cinnamon, cloves and water in a saucepan (select one large enough to hold the apples). Bring to the boil, then reduce the heat and cover the pan. Simmer the spices gently for 15 minutes, then remove from the heat. Add the lemon rind and juice and leave to stand for 15 minutes.

Meanwhile, peel, core and slice the apples, adding them to the pan as they are prepared. Add the sugar and heat the mixture, stirring, until the sugar has dissolved. When the syrup bubbles, reduce the heat and cover the pan. Simmer for 20–25 minutes, stirring occasionally, until the apples are pulpy. Remove the lid and cook, stirring the fruit pulp vigorously, until it is more or less smooth and reduced slightly. Remove from the heat, cover with a clean tea towel or kitchen paper (paper towels) – rather than a lid that will return condensation to the fruit – and leave to cool completely.

Discard the cinnamon and cloves, then stir in the fromage frais and divide the apple cream among four tall glasses or dishes. Chill before serving.

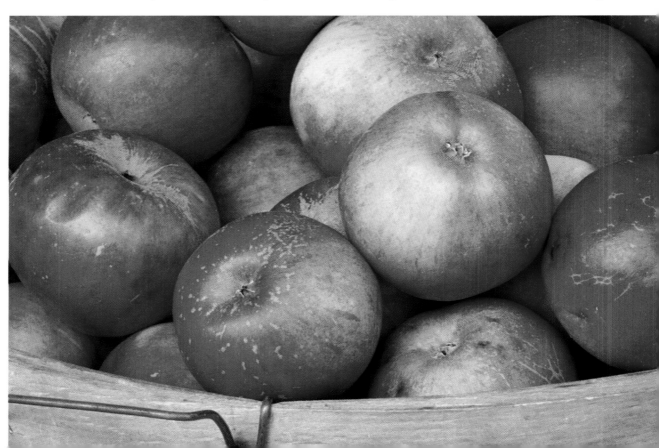

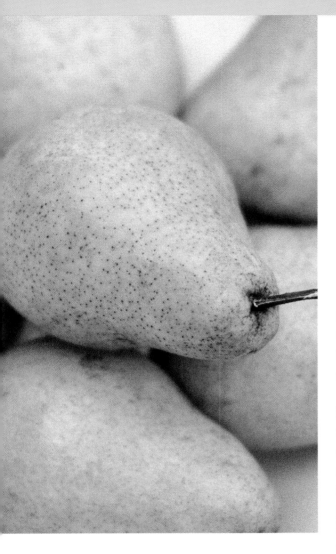

Honeyed Pears with Porridge

This is the perfect restorative breakfast – it is easy to eat and full of complex carbohydrate to provide energy until lunchtime. It is also an excellent anytime bowl of goodness for anyone lacking appetite or needing a boost to the system. Pears are easy to eat and digest, calming and a useful source of vitamins and minerals. Dressed with a honey-ginger syrup to enliven and restore, the pears can be cooked when convenient and chilled for up to 3 days, then warmed up in the microwave. While warm pears with creamy porridge induce feelings of trust and reassurance, chilled pears on steaming hot porridge bring a zingy boost of flavour and temperature contrast.

Serves 4

grated rind and juice of 1 lemon
50 g/2 oz fresh ginger root, peeled and finely chopped
300 ml/½ pint/1¼ cups water
4 firm pears
5 tablespoons honey

Porridge
900 ml/1½ pints/3¾ cups milk
175 g/6 oz/¾ cup rolled oats
½ teaspoon salt

Bring the lemon rind and juice, ginger and water to the boil in a saucepan. Reduce the heat, cover the pan and simmer for 15 minutes. Remove from the heat.

Peel, core and quarter the pears, adding them to the pan as they are ready. Add the honey and heat until simmering. Cover and cook for about 20 minutes, or until the pears are tender. Use a draining spoon to transfer the pears to a dish. Bring the honey syrup to the boil and boil, uncovered, until it is reduced by over half to a thick glaze. Pour over the pears and set aside. Cool and chill if the porridge is not being made and eaten promptly.

To make the porridge, pour the milk into a saucepan and stir in the oats and salt. Bring to the boil, stirring continuously, then reduce the heat to the minimum setting and cook, stirring occasionally, for 8–10 minutes. Divide the porridge between four bowls, then top with the pears.

Minted Blackcurrant Smoothie

Supplementing the diet with beneficial drinks is an excellent way of increasing energy and nutrient levels or bringing back the sense of purpose to life. Perhaps the feel-good factor comes from the wonderfully satisfying, virtuous and healthy feelings induced by preparing drinks.

Serves 1

50 g/2 oz/⅓ cup blackcurrants
6 mint leaves
1 tablespoon honey
300 ml/½ pint/1 cup mild yogurt
2–3 ice cubes

Whiz the blackcurrants and mint leaves with the honey in a blender until puréed. Add the yogurt and blend until smooth. Pour into a glass, add some ice cubes and serve.

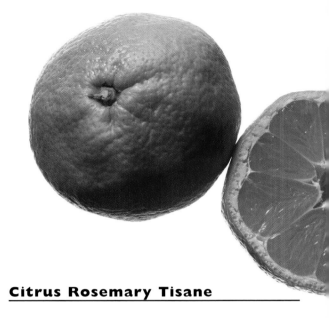

Citrus Rosemary Tisane

Stimulating lemon and warming orange are a good match for powerful rosemary, known as a stimulant and head-clearing herb and tonic. This is an excellent alternative to coffee, providing the stimulating qualities without the drawbacks of caffeine that inhibits nutrient absorption and becomes addictive. Enjoy the aroma and sip in the goodness of this warm, fruity herb drink.

Serves 1

2 rosemary sprigs
250 ml/8 fl oz/1 cup boiling water
grated rind and juice of ½ orange
grated rind and juice of ½ lemon
1–2 teaspoons honey, or to taste

Heat a mug or glass with boiling water. Place the rosemary in the mug, pour in the boiling water and cover. Leave the rosemary to infuse to about 3 minutes. Then stir in the orange and lemon rind and juice. Stir in the honey and drink warm.

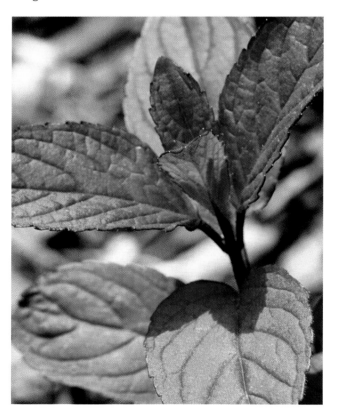

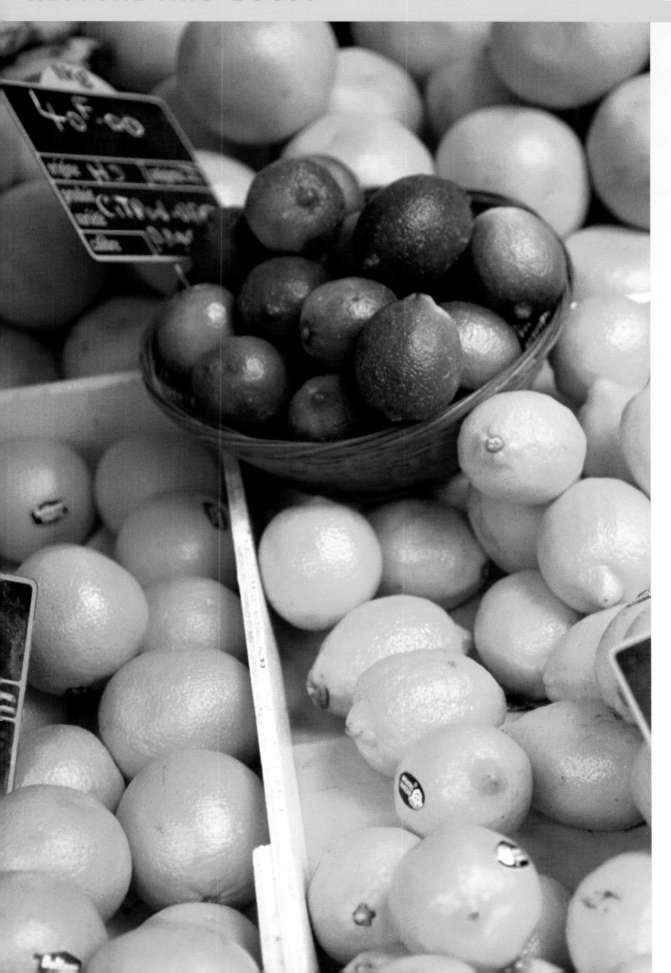

The familiar idea of comfort food is almost always associated with guilt. Well, forget all negative associations and read on. Food and eating should be comforting and reassuring when necessary – there is nothing more natural. Babies are comforted and reassured by suckling so why shouldn't these positive associations continue throughout life until, as adults, we are reassured by eating?

It is all about getting the balance right. Eating is not – and should not be – the answer to emotional problems that need tackling at source and resolving by other suitable means. Overeating is a problem, as is an ongoing dependence on food as a source of comfort, or resorting to it repeatedly as sole support in times of need. However, shopping for, preparing and cooking, and eating foods that help to create a sense of security when life is difficult can offer additional, valuable support. Meal times and situations can also be part of this positive, reassuring framework.

Nutritonally, there is every reason to eat a good mixed diet during times of stress and including plenty of complex carbohydrate that promotes a sense of calm is helpful. Taking care to eat plenty of fruit and vegetables for vitamins and minerals, with dairy produce, iron-rich protein foods and a little fat ensures that the body has all the fuel it needs. This is especially important for counteracting stress and depression, avoiding digestive disorders and boosting the body's natural defense mechanisms to fight infection when it is run down.

The focus in this chapter is on marrying good nutrition with dishes that make us feel better too. A lively, bright and light salad may be just right on an energetic day to match a sunny disposition – but it cannot compete with a steaming hot cottage pie, favourite pasta dish or fruit pudding with custard to combat a horrible cold feeling inside. These recipes are comforting and reassuring in terms of preparation, eating quality and the influence their ingredients have on the body. They may not be ideal for everyday eating, seven days a week, without additional variety but, unlike traditional high-fat, sugary indulgence dishes, there is every good reason to include them in a balanced diet on an occasional basis for the goodness they offer.

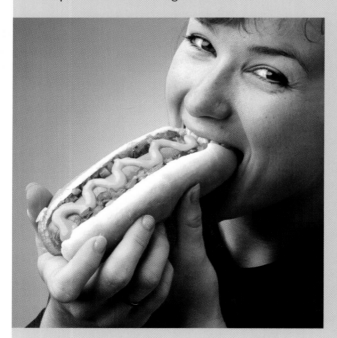

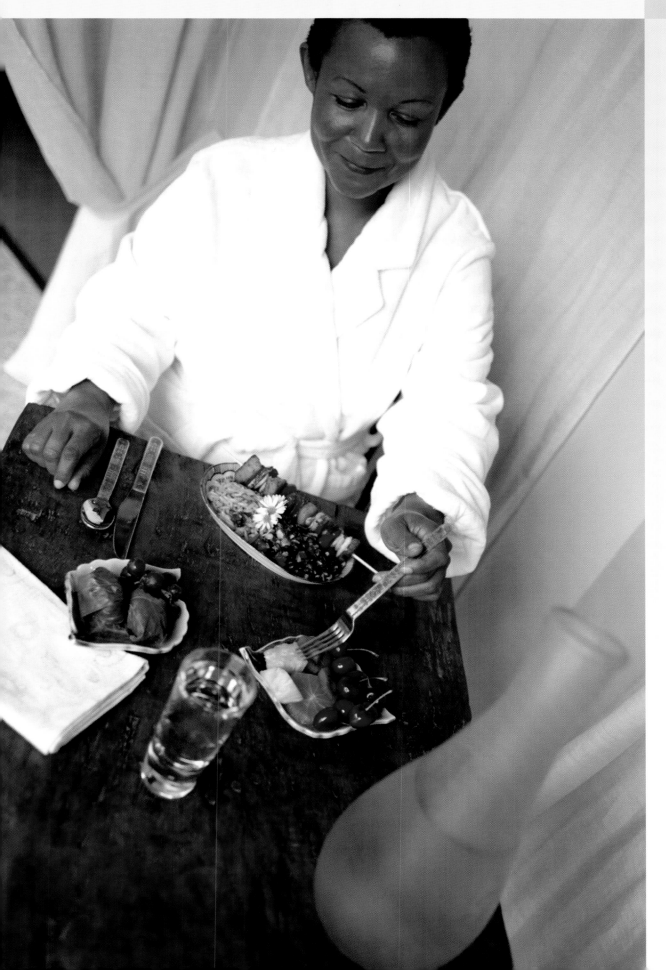

Fish Pie with Creamy Watercress Sauce and Golden Mash

Reassuring smooth textures and comforting flavours ensure that this pie rates high in the feel-good stakes. The contemporary mix of ingredients also makes it an excellent and pro-active choice to promote mental and physical wellbeing – white fish, prawns and eggs are all good for the nervous system and brain, while watercress is rich in antioxidants, vitamins and folate, and, in addition, carrots contribute beta carotene.

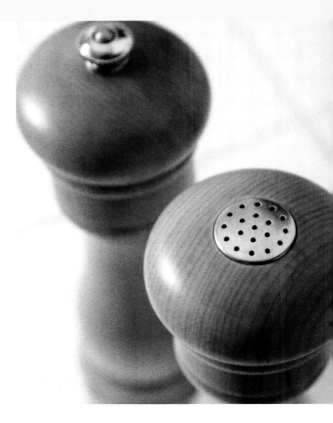

Serves 4

675 g/1½ lb potatoes, cut into chunks
225 g/8 oz carrots, thinly sliced
salt and pepper
4 tablespoons olive oil
1 small onion, chopped
2 bay leaves
2 tablespoons plain (all-purpose) flour
450 ml/¾ pint/2 cups milk
450 g/1 lb white fish fillet, skinned and cut into chunks
225 g/8 oz peeled cooked prawns (shrimp), thawed and drained if frozen
1 bunch watercress, finely chopped
grated rind of 1 lemon
2 hard-boiled eggs, roughly chopped
25 g/1 oz/⅓ cup Cheddar cheese, grated
1 thick slice wholemeal breadcrumbs

Place the potatoes and carrots in a saucepan and pour in just enough water to cover them. Add a little salt and bring to the boil. Reduce the heat, cover the pan and cook for 20 minutes, or until the vegetables are tender. Drain, reserving the water, then mash the potatoes and carrots. Stir in half the olive oil with pepper to taste.

Preheat the oven to 190°C/4375°F/Gas 5. Heat the remaining olive oil in a saucepan and add the onion and bay leaves. Stir, then cover the pan and cook over medium heat for 15 minutes, until the onion has softened. Stir in the flour to make a paste, then gradually pour in the milk and 150 ml/¼ pint/⅔ cup of the reserved cooking water. Bring to the boil, stirring continuously, then remove from heat.

Season the sauce to taste, then add the fish, prawns, watercress, lemon and eggs. Pour the mixture into a deep ovenproof dish. Top with the mashed potatoes and carrots, spreading out the vegetables evenly to cover the fish in sauce completely.

Mix the cheese and breadcrumbs and sprinkle the mixture over the top of the pie. Bake for 25–30 minutes, or until the crumb topping is crisp and golden and the pie is cooked through. Allow to stand for 5 minutes before serving.

Sardines on Toast

Serves 2

Do you remember sardines on toast? Have you ever thought of them as comfort food? If not, try this recipe and you will be converted. The problem with comfort food is that there is a tendency to fixate on the sticky chocolate puddings or the super-stodgy or fatty pastry items. Instead of always going for the obvious, seek out those illusively simple flavour combinations that may seem unlikely sources of reassurance – you may be surprised at just how soothing familiar savouries can be. Comfort yourself with the fact that this sort of old-fashioned snack brings lots of contemporary goodness by way of omega-3 fatty acids, minerals and B vitamins from fish and complex carbohydrate from the good, thick bread to bring a real mental and physical boost. A whack of garlic and zing of fresh lemon contribute a feel-good sensation. What's more, this is easy to make and lip-smackingly good.

100 g/4 oz can sardines in olive oil
salt and pepper
grated rind and juice of ½ lemon
1 garlic clove, crushed
2 large thick slices wholemeal or seeded wholegrain bread

Preheat the grill (broiler). Mash the sardines with the oil from the can. Add seasoning, the lemon rind and juice, and the garlic. When smooth and thoroughly combined, taste the sardine mixture to ensure it is perfectly seasoned.

Grill the bread on one side until browned. Spread the sardine mixture on the other side and replace under the grill. Cook until golden, then serve at once.

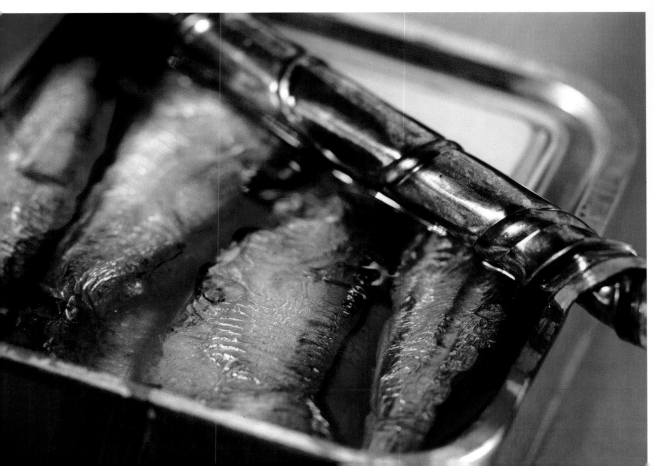

Simple Chicken, Leek and Broccoli Sauce

Making a simple chicken and mushroom sauce is gentle, traditional cooking at a basic practical level, especially when diced chicken is readily available from the supermarket. Familiar sage, parsley and thyme reassure and lift the spirits. The sauce may be served in many ways – at its simplest just ladled over pasta or into baked potatoes.

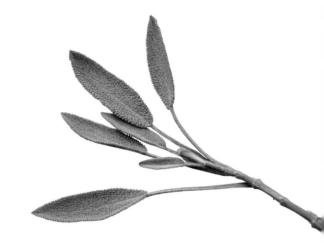

Serves 2

225 g/8 oz broccoli florets
salt and pepper
2 tablespoons olive oil
225 g/8 oz skinless boneless chicken breast, diced
4 large fresh sage leaves
2 thyme sprigs
2 leeks, sliced
2 tablespoons plain flour
250 ml/8 fl oz/1 cup milk
4 tablespoons chopped parsley

Place the broccoli in a saucepan and pour in just enough boiling water to cover the florets. Add a little salt and bring back to a full boil. Drain the broccoli, reserving the water.

Heat the oil in a large saucepan and cook the chicken, stirring, until it is just opaque. Add the sage, thyme and leeks. Stir well, then cover and cook over medium heat for 15 minutes, until the leeks are greatly reduced and softened.

Stir in the flour, then pour in 200 ml/7 fl oz/ ¾ cup of the reserved broccoli cooking water and the milk, stirring all the time. Bring to the boil, stirring. Reduce the heat, cover the pan and simmer for 10 minutes, stirring occasionally, until the chicken is cooked.

Add the broccoli and seasoning to taste. Bring back to the boil and simmer gently for a further 3–5 minutes, until the broccoli is just tender. Stir in the parsley, check the seasoning and serve.

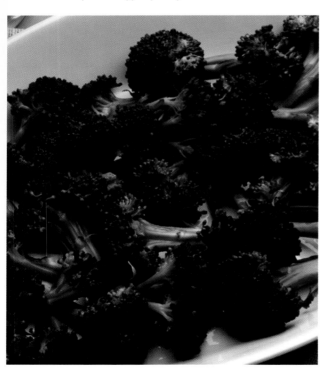

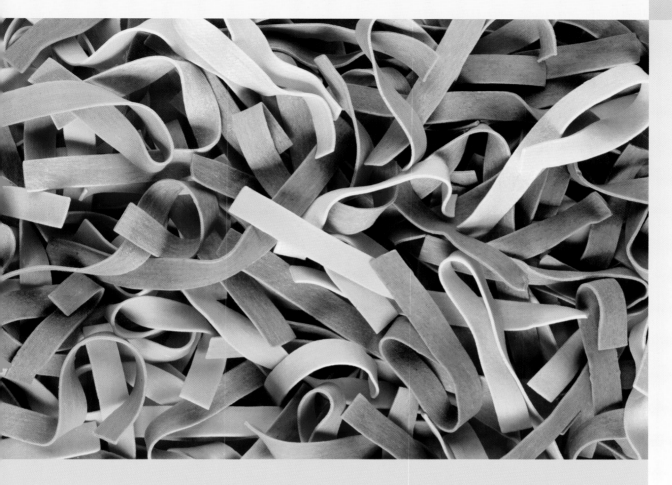

Serving Suggestions

- Ladle the sauce over spaghetti or pasta shapes.

- Spoon the sauce into large, fluffy baked potatoes.

- Serve the sauce on couscous tossed with a little grated lemon rind and warmed olive oil or melted butter.

- Use the sauce as a base for a delicious potato-topped pie – make the mashed potatoes and carrots from the Fish Pie (page 140) recipe. Do not cook the sauce once the broccoli is added (it will finish cooking in the oven). Turn the sauce into an ovenproof dish and top with the potato. Dot with butter and brown in the oven at 200°C/400°F/ Gas 6 for about 15 minutes.

- The sauce is delicious in lasagne: use 300 ml/½ pint/1 cup cooking liquid from the broccoli and 300 ml/½ pint/1 cup milk. Layer the thin sauce with no-need-to-precook lasagne in a well-greased ovenproof dish, starting with a layer of lasagne and ending with a layer of sauce. Sprinkle with wholemeal breadcrumbs mixed with some freshly grated Parmesan cheese and bake at 180°C/350°F/Gas 4 for about 40 minutes, or until the top is golden. Allow to stand for 10 minutes before cutting and serving.

Cottage Pie

The aroma, appearance, texture and flavours in this classic dish are all conducive to comfort and reassurance. The smooth, creamy and carbohydrate-packed mashed potato is absolutely perfect with the rich, meaty sauce. The hint of crispness on the crust emphasizes the overall moistness of the pie that looks simple and appealing, and fulfils every expectation. Enjoy making this pie and go for only the best, with plenty of gravy and lots of topping to seal in all the flavours underneath. Serve with lots of buttery, stir-fried cabbage.

Serves 4–6

2 tablespoons sunflower oil
500 g/1¼ lb good quality minced beef
1 large onion, chopped
2 bay leaves
2 teaspoons dried thyme
2 large carrots, diced
225 g/8 oz mushrooms, roughly chopped
salt and pepper
2 tablespoons plain flour
600 ml/1 pint/2½ cups water
dash of Worcestershire sauce
good handful of parsley, chopped

Topping
1.5 kg/3 lb potatoes
50 g/2 oz/¼ cup butter
a little milk

Heat the oil in a large heavy saucepan or flameproof casserole. Add the minced beef and brown it over fairly high heat, stirring more or less continuously. When the meat is well browned, use a draining spoon to transfer it to a bowl and set aside.

Reduce the heat slightly and add the onion, bay leaves, thyme and carrots to the fat remaining in the pan. Cook, stirring, for about 10 minutes, until the vegetables are beginning to brown. Then stir in the mushrooms with salt and pepper to taste. Cook over medium heat, stirring often, until the excess liquor from the mushrooms has evaporated.

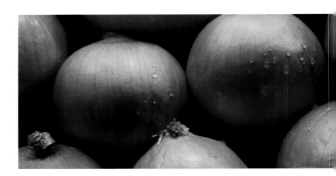

Replace the minced beef, with any juices that may have seeped from it, and stir in the flour. Add the water and a jolly good dash of Worcestershire sauce. Sprinkle in a little seasoning and bring to the boil. As soon as the mixture boils, reduce the heat so that it barely simmers. Cover and cook for 45 minutes, until the beef is tender and the sauce well flavoured. Taste for seasoning, stir in the parsley and remove from the heat.

Meanwhile, cook the potatoes in boiling salted water for about 20 minutes, or until tender. Preheat the oven to 200°C/400°F/Gas 6. Drain and mash the potatoes, adding two-thirds of the butter, plenty of freshly ground pepper (preferably white – it tastes fabulous in mashed potato) and enough milk to make the potato just soft enough to spread. Do not make the mash too sloppy or it will not absorb the glorious meat gravy.

Turn the meat mixture into a deep ovenproof dish. (If it has been cooked in a suitable flameproof casserole you may be able to leave it where it is.) Top with the potato. There is an art to adding the potato without making the meaty gravy bubble up into a mess: use a spoon to place smallish dollops of potato all around the edge of the dish, starting at opposite points. Then add dollops in the middle. Before adding any more potato, use a fork to drag the edge of the potato gently up to the dish so that it seals in the meat. Then gently drag the edges of the dollops together without pressing the potato down. Finally (sounds more tiresome than it is – this is quite therapeutic, really), add the rest of the potato in small dollops, evenly all over the top of the pie and spread it evenly with a fork.

Dot the top with the remaining butter and bake for 30–40 minutes, until crisp and golden. Allow the cottage pie to stand for 10 minutes before serving.

Pork, Lamb or Poultry Pie

Minced pork, lamb, chicken or turkey can be used instead of beef in the cottage pie. The flavour may be different, but the essential combination of textures is still superlative.

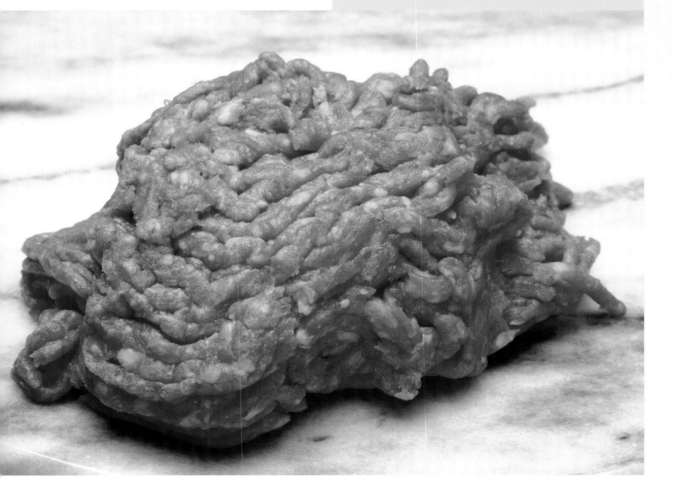

Succulent Lamb Hotpot with Herb Dumplings

No section on comfort food would be complete without a meaty stew and fluffy dumplings. And this is just that: a moist, rich stew full of goodness from lean lamb and a little kidney for excellent flavour, with tender carrots and juicy small whole onions. The dumplings are quite special – flavoured with tarragon, thyme and parsley and then baked on the open casserole, they develop a golden crust on top that contrasts with their moist bases and fluffy middles.

Serves 4

500 g/1¼ lb lean boneless lamb, cubed
2 lamb's kidneys, cored and finely diced
2 tablespoons plain (all-purpose) flour
salt and pepper
2 tablespoons sunflower oil
450 g/1 lb pickling onions
4 carrots, diced
2 bay leaves
900 ml/1½ pints/3¾ cups lamb or chicken stock

Dumplings
225 g/8 oz/2 cups self-raising flour (all-purpose flour with baking powder)
100 g/4 oz/½ cup shredded suet
4 tablespoons chopped parsley
1 tablespoon chopped tarragon
1 tablespoon chopped thyme
175 ml/6 fl oz/¾ cup cold water

Preheat the oven to 160°C/325°F/Gas 3. In a bowl, mix the lamb and kidney with the flour and plenty of seasoning. Toss the meats in the flour until evenly coated. Heat the sunflower oil in a large frying pan (skillet). Brown the lamb and kidney all over, then use a draining spoon to transfer the meats to a large, deep casserole. Do this in two batches.

Fry the onions until they are browned all over, then add them to the meats. Cook the carrots and bay leaves in the same fat for a few minutes, then pour in the stock and stir until it comes to the boil. Pour the carrots, stock and bay leaves over the lamb, scraping all residue from the pan. Add seasoning, stir well and cover.

Cook in the oven for 2 hours, stirring occasionally, until the meat is succulent and the cooking liquor full flavoured. Check to ensure that the stew is barely simmering rather than cooking too rapidly as there should be plenty of liquid left for cooking the dumplings once the meat is tender. Remove the casserole from the oven and increase the temperature to 180°C/350°F/Gas 4.

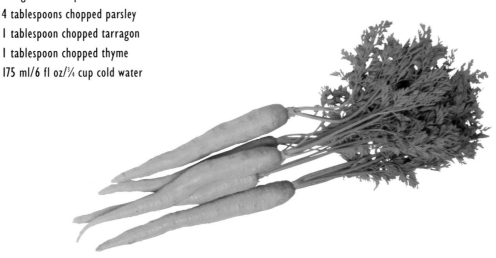

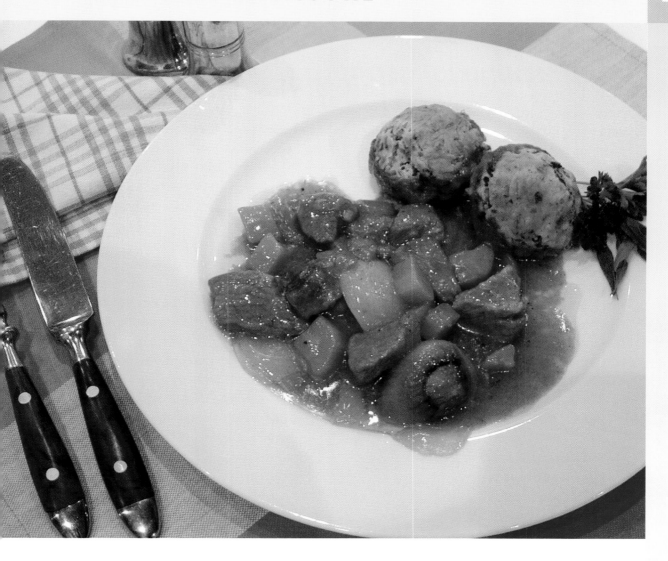

To make the dumplings, mix the flour, suet, parsley and thyme in a bowl. Add a good pinch of salt, then mix in the water to make a soft, but not too sticky, dough. Cut the dough in half, then cut each half into quarters to make eight portions. Place a spoonful of flour on the work surface and shape a portion of dough into a neat ball. Shape the remaining portions into balls to make neat round dumplings.

Stir the stew and make sure there is lots of liquid left – there should be plenty if the stew was cooking gently rather than boiling. Place the dumplings on top of the casserole and put it back in the oven. Bake, uncovered, for 30–40 minutes, until the dumplings are risen, browned and lightly crisped on top. Lift one dumpling from the pot to check whether it is cooked – the underneath should be moist and glossy, and the middle fluffy. Serve at once.

Beef Stew

The recipe works equally well with beef. Use leg or shin of beef for a fabulous flavour, with beef stock instead of lamb, and increase the cooking time to 2½ or 3 hours initially, depending on how tender the beef is.

Pork and Vegetable Hash

Hash conjures all sorts of images, good or bad depending on childhood associations or previous experience of the dish. This fresh, modern version is deliciously full of flavour and food value, and wonderfully comforting to eat. Making it is also one of those pleasurable cooking experiences, a time for grating root vegetables and stirring ingredients that smell wonderful as they cook. This will have everyone running to the kitchen waiting to share a suppertime experience. Serve large bowls of watercress sprigs and little cherry tomatoes as accompaniments so that they can be eaten with the fingers to complement the hash and cleanse the palate.

Serves 4

2 tablespoons sunflower oil
1 large onion, chopped
2 garlic cloves, crushed
2 large carrots, coarsely grated
1 small parsnip, grated
1 large raw or cooked beetroot, peeled and grated
450 g/1 lb potatoes, coarsely grated
450 g/1 lb lean minced pork
salt and pepper
handful of parsley, chopped
6 large sage leaves, shredded
50 g/2 oz/1 cup fresh wholemeal breadcrumbs
1 egg

Heat the oil in a large non-stick frying pan (skillet). Add the onion, garlic, carrots, parsnip, beetroot if using raw, and potatoes. Stir well, cover and cook for 5 minutes.

Stir in the pork with plenty of salt and pepper and cook until it is thoroughly combined with the vegetables, then remove the pan from the heat. Add the parsley, sage and breadcrumbs. Beat the egg and add it to the pan, then mix well until all the ingredients are thoroughly mixed together.

Press the mixture down evenly in the pan and replace it over low to medium heat. Cook for 20–30 minutes, until the base of the hash is well browned. At this stage there are two options: either place the pan of hash under the grill (broiler) on a moderate setting and cook until it is well browned all over, or place a large plate over the hash and invert the pan and plate. Remove the pan, add and heat a little more oil, if necessary, then slide the hash back into the pan. Cook until the hash is golden underneath and cooked through. Serve cut into wedges.

Cooked Meat and Vegetable Hash

Make a fabulously simple hash using leftover cooked potatoes, carrots, parsnips, swedes (rutabagas), cabbage or any other vegetables. Place them in a big bowl and chop at them with a knife to part mash and bind, part dice or chop them until they cling together. Add chopped or diced leftover cooked meat or poultry, or canned corned beef or cooked ham. Flavour with chopped fresh herbs and seasoning to taste. Heat a little oil in a frying pan (skillet) and turn the mixture into it, then press it down evenly and firmly. Cook for about 15 minutes, until well browned underneath. Brush with oil and finish cooking under a hot grill. Delicious!

Bacon Sandwiches with Glorious Pepper Salad

Bacon sandwiches always seem to bring back memories – early morning stop-offs on important journeys, lazy weekend breakfasts, or snatched lunches at unlikely cafés. The appetite-arousing smell of bacon cooking is reassuring and spirit lifting – it is perfect comfort food and especially good in

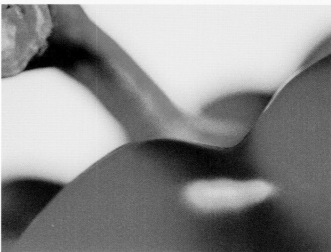

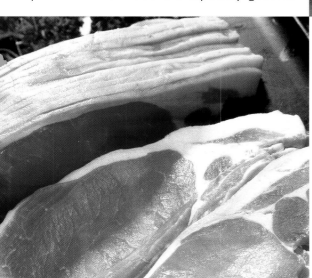

thick chunks of seeded or wholemeal bread with lots of just-off-crunchy vegetables. Indulge yourself and everyone around you with these vitamin, protein and mineral-packed sandwiches.

Serves 1

2–3 rindless bacon rashers (slices)
a little olive oil
¼ tsp fennel seeds (optional)
1 red (bell) pepper, seeded and cut into strips
2 spring onions (scallions), cut into short lengths
2 thick slices wholemeal or seeded wholegrain bread
a little tomato ketchup (optional)
thin slice of white cabbage

Have a warm plate ready for the cooked bacon. Place the bacon rashers in a non-stick frying pan (skillet). Cook until they are browned on one side, then turn and cook the second side, pressing the rashers on to the pan so that they are crisped and browned. By this time, the bacon should have yielded its liquor and fat.

Use a slice to remove the bacon from the pan, setting it aside on a warm plate. Trickle a little oil into the pan if necessary, then add the fennel seeds and pepper strips. Toss the peppers for a few seconds, then add the spring onions and toss them for a few seconds too. Remove the pan from the heat.

Spread a slice of bread with a little ketchup, if using, then top with the peppers and onions. Add the slice of white cabbage, separating the shreds that overhang and tucking them back on top, and the bacon rashers. Top with the second slice of bread and serve at once.

Soothing Parsley and Sage Mash with Avocado and Bacon Topping

This is a contemporary take on comfort food, with all the warmth of creamy mash that is aromatic with soothing parsley, sage and fruity olive oil. The topping combines exciting contrasts of texture and flavour from silky avocado with crisp bacon, tender baby spinach and crunchy Iceberg lettuce and croûtons.

Serves 2

1 kg/2¼ lb potatoes
salt and pepper
6 tablespoons olive oil
4 rindless bacon rashers (slices), diced
1 garlic clove, sliced
1 thick slice seeded wholemeal, rye or Granary bread, diced
100 ml/4 fl oz crème fraîche
large handful of parsley, finely chopped
8 large sage leaves, finely shredded
bunch of chives, finely snipped
100 g/4 oz baby spinach leaves
wedge of Iceberg lettuce, finely shredded
2 spring onions (scallions), finely sliced
1 large ripe avocado, halved, pitted, peeled and diced
grated rind of 1 lemon
lemon wedges to serve

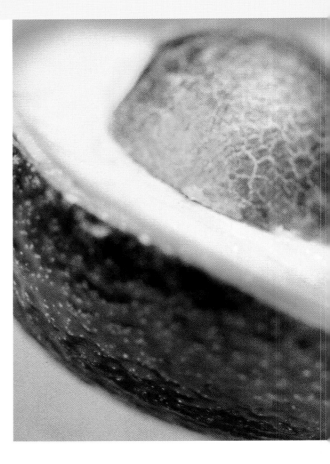

Cook the potatoes in boiling salted water for about 20 minutes, until tender. While the potatoes are cooking, heat 2 tablespoons of the oil in a frying pan (skillet) and cook the bacon until browned and crisp. Use a draining spoon to remove the bacon from the pan. Add the garlic and diced bread and cook, stirring frequently, until the bread dice are turned into crisp and golden croûtons. Set aside with the bacon.

Drain and mash the potatoes with the remaining olive oil. Stir in the crème fraîche, parsley, sage and chives. Taste for seasoning.

Mix the spinach, lettuce, spring onions, avocado and lemon rind in a bowl. Divide potato between two large bowls, hollowing out the middle. Pile the avocado salad on the potato and top with the bacon and croûtons. Garnish with lemon wedges and serve at once.

Banana, Apple and Blackcurrant Crumble

Hot puddings are dishes that everyone denounces as disaster areas for healthy eating but this proves they can be brilliantly good for you. It is the dream comfort pudding – hot and fruity, satisfyingly full of excellent slow-energy-release carbohydrate and vitamins, plus lots of useful minerals from the fruit. And the topping is full of oats, nuts and seeds, valued for their calming influences. Served with cream, low-fat fromage frais or crème fraîche, or flowing custard, this is a truly heartwarming dessert.

Serves 4

450 g/1 lb cooking apples, peeled, cored and sliced
2 small, firm bananas, thickly sliced
225 g/8 oz/2 cups blackcurrants, strung
50 g/2 oz/⅓ cup soft (light) brown sugar

Crumble Topping
50 g/2 oz/4 tablespoons butter
100 g/4 oz/1 cup plain (all-purpose) flour
100 g/4 oz/⅛ cup rolled oats
4 tablespoons sunflower seeds
4 tablespoons sesame seeds
100 g/4 oz/⅛ cup walnuts, chopped
25 g/1 oz/1 tablespoon soft (light) brown sugar

Preheat the oven to 190°C/375°F/Gas 5. Mix the apples, bananas and blackcurrants with the sugar in a large, deep ovenproof dish.

For the topping, rub the butter into the flour, either using your fingertips or in a food processor. Stir in the oats, sunflower and sesame seeds, walnuts and sugar. Sprinkle this topping over the fruit and spread it out evenly without pressing it down too firmly.

Bake the crumble for 40–45 minutes, until the topping is crisp and golden and the fruit tender. Allow to stand for 10 minutes before serving.

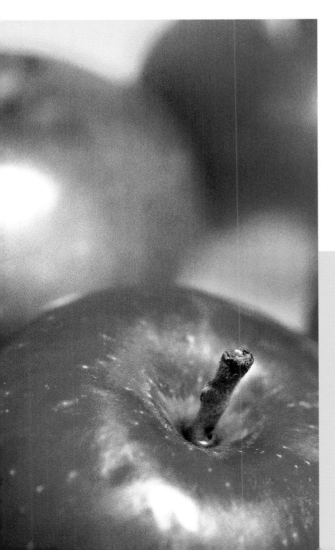

Other Fruit Combinations

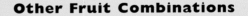

- Rhubarb with chopped candied ginger and banana.

- Cranberry and apple.

- Gooseberry with dried apricots.

Baked Rice Pudding

This classic pudding is so simple to make and very soothing to eat. Treat yourself and others to its pure simplicity, either hot or chilled, or make it a little special by following some of the suggestions at the end of the recipe.

Serves 4

40 g/1½ oz/⅓ cup pudding rice
grated rind of 1 lemon
2 tablespoons sugar
600 ml/1 pint/2½ cups milk
25 g/1 oz butter
a little freshly grated nutmeg

Preheat the oven to 160°C/325°F/Gas 3. Place the rice in a saucepan and add plenty of cold water. Bring to the boil, give the rice a stir, then drain it in a sieve and transfer it to an ovenproof dish.

Add the lemon rind, sugar and milk. Stir well and add the butter. Bake the rice for 2 hours, stirring twice. Sprinkle with a little nutmeg and bake for a further 30 minutes, until the pudding is thick and creamy, and browned on top.

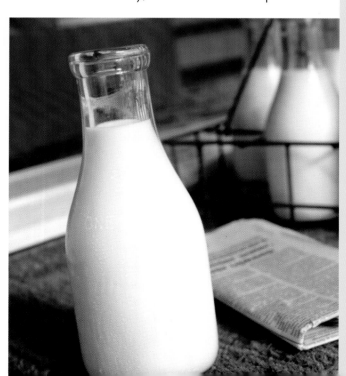

Serving Suggestions

For a creamy pudding without a baked crust, stir the pudding frequently during the last 30 minutes of cooking, scraping the edge of the mixture from the dish to prevent it from browning and forming a crust. With or without a crust, the following serving suggestions are healthy and soothing.

- For an old-fashioned nursery pudding, add a handful of sultanas (golden raisins) or raisins halfway through cooking.

- Serve the pudding chilled, layered with a mixture of summer fruit drizzled with a little maple syrup.

- Stir the pudding instead of allowing it to brown, then cool and chill it. Half-fill individual flameproof dishes with strawberries and top with the cold pudding. Cover the surface generously with sugar, pressing it into an even layer. Cook under a hot grill (broiler) until the sugar has caramelized. Cool and chill before serving.

- Swirl a little chocolate hazelnut spread into the hot pudding.

- Pan-fry peeled, cored and quartered pears in a little butter until golden and sprinkle with soft brown sugar. Cook briefly until the sugar has dissolved, then serve the pears on the hot pudding.

- Sprinkle halved and pitted peaches with sugar and brown them under a preheated grill (broiler). Serve topped with hot rice pudding.

Baked Chocolate Chip Pudding with Dark Chocolate Sauce

For many, chocolate is the ultimate comfort food. This pudding is not lusciously naughty but simply very nice. Good enough for the occasional treat with dark chocolate sauce.

Serves 6

100 g/4 oz butter
100 g/4 oz soft (light) brown sugar
1 teaspoon natural vanilla essence (extract)
2 eggs
176 g/6 oz self-raising (all-purpose) flour
4 tablespoons cocoa powder
100 g/4 oz dark chocolate cooking chips

Dark Chocolate Sauce
225 g/8 oz plain chocolate
6 tablespoons golden syrup (light corn syrup)

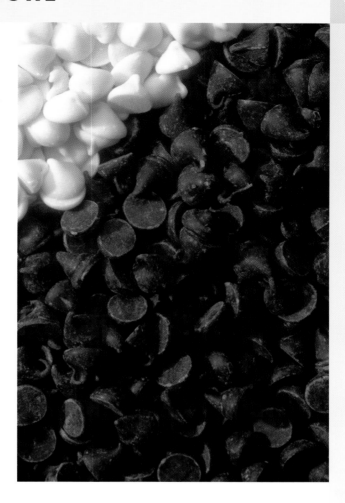

Preheat the oven to 160 C/325 F/Gas 3 and grease a 1.12 litre/2 pint ovenproof basin. Cream the butter and sugar until pale and fluffy, then beat in the vanilla. Add the eggs and a spoonful of the flour and beat the eggs into the mixture until well combined. Add the remaining flour and cocoa, and fold in the dry ingredients using a metal spoon. Fold in the chocolate cooking chips.

Turn the mixture into the prepared basin and stand it on a baking tray or tin to make it easier to slide on and off the oven shelf. Bake for 50–60 minutes, until the sponge is well risen and springy to the touch.

For the chocolate sauce, break the chocolate into pieces and place in a heatproof bowl. Add the golden syrup. Stand the bowl over a saucepan of barely simmering water and stir until the chocolate has melted and thoroughly combined with the syrup.

Slide a flexible spatula around the inside of the basin and down as far as possible to loosen the pudding, then invert it on to a plate. Cut the pudding into wedges and serve with the chocolate sauce.

Steamed Lemon Sponge Pudding with Warm Lemon Curd

This moist, citrus-scented sponge pudding is topped with freshly made lemon curd. Serve it with creamy custard for an appealingly comforting pudding. There are plenty of alternatives to the lemon curd, and softly whipped cream or thick Greek-style yogurt may be served instead of custard.

Serves 6

100 g/4 oz/½ cup butter
100 g/4 oz/⅔ cup soft (light) brown sugar
grated rind and juice of 1 lemon
2 eggs
176 g/6 oz/1⅓ cup self-raising (all-purpose) flour

Lemon Curd Sauce
1 large egg, beaten
grated rind and juice of 1 large lemon
100 g/4 oz/⅔ cup castor (fine) sugar
40 g/1½ oz/1½ tablespoons unsalted butter, diced

Prepare a large saucepan and steamer, and grease a 1.12 litre/2 pint/5 cup basin. Cream the butter and sugar until pale and fluffy, then beat in the lemon rind. Add the eggs and a spoonful of the flour and beat the eggs into the mixture until well combined. Fold in the remaining flour using a metal spoon, then fold in the lemon juice.

Turn the mixture into the basin and cover with a piece of pleated greaseproof (waxed) paper. Top with double-thick pleated foil, crumpling it tightly around the rim of the basin to prevent steam from entering. If the basin has a thick rim, then it may be easier to tie the foil in place with string. (The pleat in the paper and foil allow the covering to expand as the pudding mixture rises during cooking.)

Steam the pudding for 1¾–2 hours, or until it is risen and firm to the touch. Check the water level in the pan under the steamer regularly to make sure it does not boil dry during cooking.

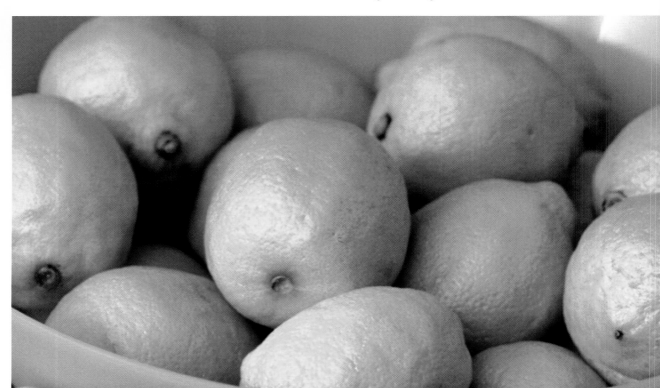

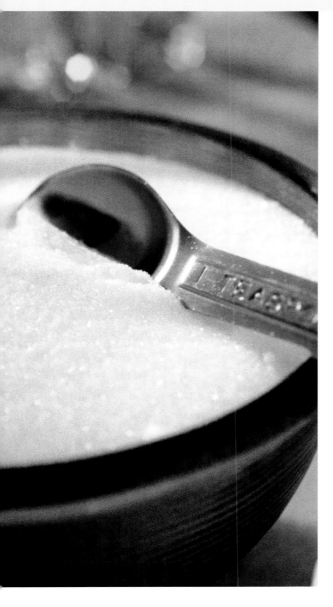

Make the lemon curd sauce so that it will be ready shortly before the pudding is cooked. Beat the egg with the lemon rind and juice and sugar in a heatproof bowl. Add the butter and stand the bowl over a saucepan of hot, not simmering, water. The water should be kept just below simmering point – if it begins to simmer or boil, the mixture will overcook and curdle quickly. Stir the mixture until the butter has melted completely and the curd thickened enough to coat the back of a spoon – this takes about 20 minutes. Remove the bowl from the saucepan.

Use a flexible spatula to loosen the pudding from the basin, sliding it all around the rim and down to the base. Invert the pudding on to a serving dish and pour the warm lemon curd over the top. Serve at once, with a hot custard sauce.

Simple Custard Sauce

This is a simple custard which is stabilized with cornflour, which prevents it from curdling. The flavour and texture is lighter than and superior to 'convenience' sauce made with commercial custard powder.

Mix 1 tablespoon cornflour and 2 tablespoons sugar with 4 egg yolks and 1–2 teaspoons natural vanilla essence (extract). The amount of vanilla depends on type – the better type with bourbon is delicate and can be used in larger amounts. If the essence smells harsh and strong, use 1 teaspoon or less and add more when the sauce is cooked, if necessary. Stir in a little milk taken from 600 ml/1 pint. Heat the remaining milk to just below boiling point, then stir it into the cornflour and yolk mixture. Pour the mixture back into the saucepan and bring to the boil, stirring continuously, over low to medium heat. When the custard boils and thickens, remove the pan from the heat and serve at once.

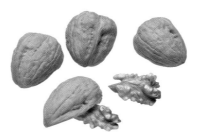